BASIC FACTS IN
ORTHOPAEDICS

. . . and set me down in the midst of the valley which was full of bones.

. . . behold there were very many in the open valley; and, lo, they were very dry.

Thus saith the Lord God unto these bones; Behold I will cause breath to enter into you, and ye shall live:

And I will lay sinews upon you and will bring flesh upon you and cover you with skin, and put breath in you, and ye shall live.

Ezekiel 37.

BASIC FACTS IN ORTHOPAEDICS

PATRICK S. H. BROWNE
MA, BM, BCh, FRCS
Senior Lecturer in Orthopaedics
University of Tasmania

BLACKWELL
SCIENTIFIC PUBLICATIONS
OXFORD LONDON EDINBURGH
BOSTON MELBOURNE

© 1981 by
Blackwell Scientific Publications
Editorial offices:
Osney Mead, Oxford, OX2 0EL
8 John Street, London, WC1N 2ES
9 Forrest Road, Edinburgh,
    EH1 2QH
52 Beacon Street, Boston
    Massachusetts 02108, USA
214 Berkeley Street, Carlton
    Victoria 3053, Australia

First published 1981

Typeset by Scottish Studios and
Engravers Ltd, Glasgow.
Printed and bound in Great Britain
by Billing & Sons Ltd.,
Guildford, Worcester and London

DISTRIBUTORS

USA
    Blackwell Mosby Book
    Distributors, 11830 Westline
    Industrial Drive, St Louis,
    Missouri 63141

Canada
    Blackwell Mosby Book
    Distributors, 120 Melford Drive,
    Scarborough, Ontario,
    M1B 2X4

Australia
    Blackwell Scientific Book
    Distributors, 214 Berkeley
    Street, Carlton, Victoria 3053

British Library
Cataloguing in Publication Data
Browne, Patrick S. H.
    Basic facts in orthopaedics
    1. Orthopedia
    I. Title
    617'.3   RD731
    ISBN 0–632–00718–4

Contents

Preface

Medical students are taught many things. So much is taught that it is almost beyond the capacity of the average student to learn it all. More intelligent and more intellectual students are being recruited.

The average student has the capacity to become the average doctor—whose qualities of patience, integrity and good-humoured durability appeal to the average patient. The more intelligent and more intellectual doctor may not have these qualities.

The basic facts of orthopaedics are explicable to the average student—the minutiae of orthopaedic practice may not be. There are differences of opinion even among orthopaedic surgeons concerning the minutiae.

This book is written for the average medical student in the hope that it will help him in his struggle to become the average doctor.

I thank all those who have helped with this book. In particular I thank Mrs Hilary Goldsmid for the excellence of her illustrations.

P.S.H.B.

CHAPTER 1

Adult Bone

Bone is composed of an organic matrix known as osteoid. This consists of collagen fibres embedded in a cementing gel of protein polysaccharide. A mineral known as apatite consisting of calcium and phosphate is deposited on the collagen fibres as needle-shaped crystals.

In adult bone the collagen fibres are aligned to parallel the average compression and tension stresses to which the bone is subject. The apatite crystals are similarly orientated on the collagen fibres.

The strength of bones is dependent both on the normal formation of osteoid and mineral and on this alignment parallel to the average stresses to which the bone is subject.

Long bones in adults consist of tubes of cortical bone. The hollow centre contains marrow and occasional trabeculae of cancellous bone. The ends of bone are expanded towards the articular surface. This expansion is the metaphysis – here the cortex is thinned but arcades of cancellous bone supporting the articular surface are more pronounced (Fig. 1.1). These arcades also parallel the average stress to which the ends of the bone is subject and are aligned to transmit these stresses to the diaphysis (Fig. 1.2).

The shaft of a long bone is ensheathed in a layer of periosteum. The outer portion of this layer is fibrous tissue; the inner portion (cambium) contains primitive mesenchymal cells. The lining of the marrow cavity is known as endosteum and also is a source of primitive mesenchymal cells.

Pluripotent mesenchymal cells are present in the periosteum and the endosteum and also the trabeculae. They can develop into:

1. Osteoblasts which lay down new bone.

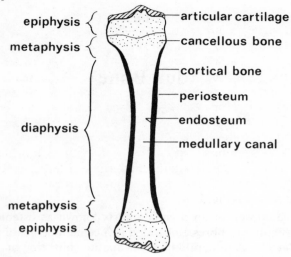

Fig. 1.1   Parts of bone.

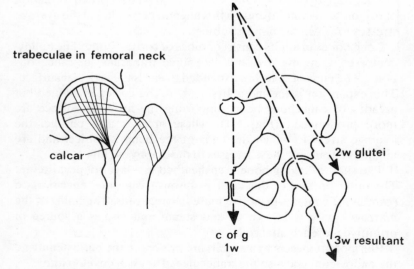

Fig. 1.2   Trabeculae aligned along the lines of stress; w, body weight.

2. Osteoclasts which reabsorb bone.

This activity is stimulated by trauma (fracture) or by infection or tumours which tend to displace the periosteum. These lesions cause a periosteal reaction which are visible on radiographs as new bone.

The cortex of a long bone is made of well-organised compact bone. This bone is organised in a series of Haversian systems (each an osteon) based on a central blood vessel. Osteocytes are embedded in the bone surrounding the blood vessel and are joined to it by minute canaliculi. The osteocytes maintain bone and are associated with its biochemical turnover. The alignment of the lamellae of each osteon is slightly different from its neighbour. This varied alignment adds strength to the bone, particularly as regards tangential stresses (Fig. 1.3).

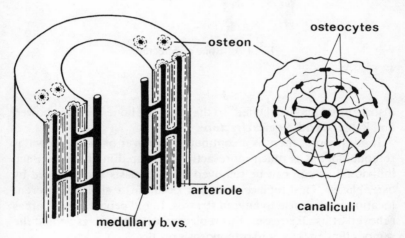

Fig. 1.3   Haversian system.

Cancellous bone is present towards the ends of long bones. The trabeculae are arranged adjacent to blood vessels; they are thinner and less complex than the lamellae of the cortex. The trabeculae are arranged to parallel the average compression and tension stresses to which the ends of bone are subject (Fig. 1.4).

Any lesion which interferes with the normal arrangement of cortical or cancellous bone will tend to weaken it. An example of such a lesion is Paget's disease in which there is no deficiency in the amount of bone. However the internal architecture of bone is

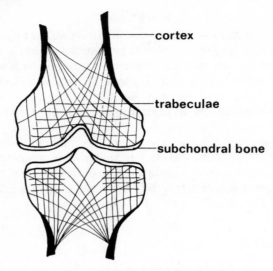

cortex

trabeculae

subchondral bone

Fig. 1.4   Bone architecture.

disorganised and weakened, so that the long bones become bowed and liable to pathological fracture.

In all people, there is a continuous turnover of bone known as remodelling. It is much more active and rapid in children. Each individual osteon can be removed by osteoclasts and replaced by osteoblasts. This replacement can occur in a slightly different location in response to altered stresses. In old people, and in areas relieved of usual stresses, this replacement process lags behind the remodelling process and osteoporosis results.

The process of remodelling:

1. Permits a micro repair mechanism for wear and tear of minor trauma. It acts as a built-in protection against 'fatigue' (in the metallurgical sense).

2. It permits realignment of lamellae in response to changes of loads.

The blood supply of an adult long bone is:

1. From a central nutrient artery which supplies the marrow endosteum and the inner two-thirds of the cortex of the diaphysis.

2. Vessels from the periosteum which supply the outer one-third of the cortex.

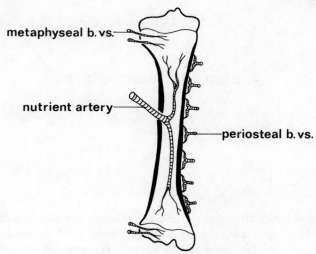

metaphyseal b. vs.

nutrient artery

periosteal b. vs.

Fig. 1.5   Blood supply to a long bone.

3. Various vessels in the metaphyseal region (Fig. 1.5).
Lesions which disrupt the blood supply to a bone will cause that part of the bone to die.

CHAPTER 2

Calcium Haemostasis

It is necessary to maintain the serum calcium ion concentration at about 10mg per cent (4.7 – 5.2 m/cg/litre) as it is involved in numerous vital functions. Bone forms a reservoir of calcium and phosphate. There is a rapid turnover between bone and the extracellular fluid in order to maintain the serum calcium. Various factors are involved in this homoestatic process.

Parathormone secretion is stimulated by lowering of the serum calcium concentration and inhibited by an increase.

1. It has the function of promoting bone reabsorption and thus raising the serum calcium.

2. It also increases the excretion of phosphate by the kidney.

Vitamin D also affects the homeostasis of calcium.

1. It promotes the absorption of calcium from the intestine.

2. It promotes the activity of parathormone on bone.

3. It promotes bone accretion in patients with Vitamin D deficiency.

Calcitonin from the thyroid lowers serum calcium ion concentration by inhibiting bone reabsorption.

The level of serum calcium is closely linked with that of phosphate. It depends on absorption from the intestine and on reabsorption from the kidney tubules. Phosphate is also excreted and reabsorbed from the kidney tubules. The level of serum calcium may be affected by alimentary and kidney lesions. These lesions will have the greatest effect in children in whom the utilisation and turnover of calcium and phosphate is so much greater.

CHAPTER 3

Epiphyseal Growth Plate

Longitudinal growth of bone in children takes place at the epiphyseal growth plate, which is a plate of cartilage between the bone of the epiphysis and that of the metaphysis in a long bone. Several zones of the plate are described (Fig. 3.1).

1. The zone of germinal and of proliferating cartilage adjacent to the epiphysis. New cartilage cells are developed here and form cartilage matrix.

2. The zone of maturing cartilage where the cells form palisades and hypertrophy.

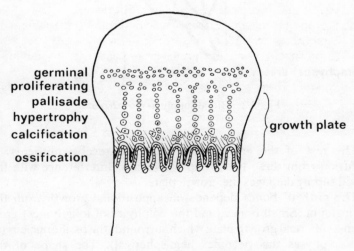

Fig. 3.1   Growth plate.

7

3. The zone of calcifying cartilage. The matrix becomes impregnated with apatite and the cells degenerate and die.

4. The zone of osteogenesis. The degenerating and dead cells are reabsorbed and are replaced by osteoblasts which secrete osteoid. The osteoid is rapidly mineralised with apatite and primitive bone results.

5. The zone of remodelling. Some of the new bone is reabsorbed as the shaft narrows and more regularly arranged lamellar bone is formed.

The growth plate has blood supply (Fig. 3.2):

1. From vessels to the epiphysis which reaches the germinal zone of cartilage.

2. From vessels to the metaphysis which reaches the area of degenerating cartilage.

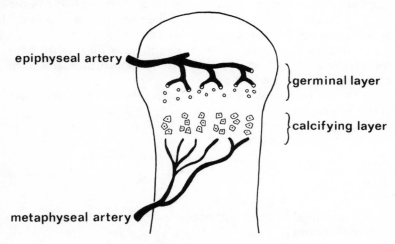

epiphyseal artery

germinal layer

calcifying layer

metaphyseal artery

Fig. 3.2   Blood supply to growth plate.

The rest of the growth plate can only receive nutrients by diffusion from these two groups of vessels. Interference with the blood supply damages the growth plate.

The girth of bones depends on appositional growth from the periosteum. Small bones (and the epiphyses of long bones) grow from a spherical growth plate which surrounds the ossific nucleus (in the epiphyses this becomes hemispherical). The shape of the epiphyses and of small bones depends very much on neighbouring contiguous structures. If the anatomy is distorted (as in club foot) the eventual shape of the bone will be distorted too.

The shape of the bone is also dependent on the stresses to which it is subject during growth. The upper end of the femur is subject to traction from its various muscle attachments. In particular, the abductor muscles (gluteus medius and minimus) and the psoas and adductors are normally in balance. In certain conditions such as meningomyelocele, cerebral palsy and poliomyelitis, the pull of the abductor muscles is relatively weak. As a result, the epiphysis of the greater trochanter does not develop fully and growth of the upper part of the femoral neck is reduced. Coxa valga results (Fig. 3.3).

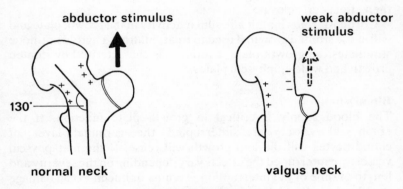

Fig. 3.3   Coxa valga.

The growth plate is affected by:
1. Nutritional factors.
2. Biochemical factors.
3. Hormones.
4. Blood supply.

Nutritional factors
Any generalised nutritional deficiency will be apparent at the growth plate as it is an area of high metabolic activity. Vitamin C is important in collagen synthesis; infantile scurvy is reflected in defects at the epiphyseal growth plate.

Biochemical factors
Calcium and phosphate are deposited as hydroxyapatite in the zone of calcifying cartilage and the zone of osteogenesis in the growth

plate. The condition known as rickets develops from defects of calcium and phosphate metabolism, in the growing child. The formation of cartilage matrix involves the production of chondroitin. Defects in mucopolysaccharide metabolism are reflected in dysfunction of the growth plate and is seen in the group of conditions known as mucopolysaccharidoses.

Hormones

Growth hormone promotes the activity of the growth plate cells; both cartilage formation and bone formation are increased. Excessive activity produces giants; deficiency produces dwarfs. Testosterone and oestrogen will stimulate the growth plate cells and then effect early closure.

Corticosteroids inhibit all cellular activity in the growth plate and will cause stunted growth if used to treat children. Thyroid hormone stimulates the growth plate. Cretinism is characterised by stunted growth and wide epiphyseal plates.

Blood supply

The blood supply is critical to growth plate function. If the epiphyseal vessels are interrupted the germinal layer of chondrocytes will die and growth will cease. If the metaphyseal vessels are interruped the effects vary depending on the severity and length of time of the interruption. Trauma or infection can damage the blood supply to the growth plate.

Generalised interference of growth plate function can produce:
1. Dwarfism.
2. Altered proportions of limbs to trunk.
3. Multiple deformities.
4. Early onset of degenerative joint disease.
5. Associated systemic manifestations.

Interference of function at one specific growth plate produces:
1. Limb length discrepancy.
2. Deformity.
3. Early onset of degenerative change in the adjacent joint.

CHAPTER 4

Leg Length Discrepancy

Many people have a discrepancy in leg lengths of about one centimetre. They can accommodate themselves to this discrepancy with no symptoms and no outward physical signs. Such people require no physical treatment.

However, leg length discrepancy can be severe and cause a limp and symptoms in the lumbar spine due to mechanical derangement. In some patients with congenital abnormalities the limbs may be so short that they will require an extension prosthesis.

CAUSES OF LEG DISCREPANCY

Congenital

There are many causes of congenital leg length discrepancy. Many of these can be classified as dysmelias (which means a failure in development of the limb). An amelia is congenital absence of the limb.

A phocomelia occurs in patients who have a flipper limb, the hand or foot extremity being attached directly onto the axial skeleton. These deformities occurred as a result of the thalidomide tragedy.

A proximal focal femoral defect occurs in various grades of severity. In this condition, the femur is deficient proximally and in the most severe form, only the distal end of the femur is apparently attached to the pelvis.

Infections

Osteomyelitis or septic arthritis in infancy may damage the epiphyseal growth plate and cause incomplete growth. Over the years, a very significant growth disturbance takes place, and the limb may be very short (particularly if the epiphysis at the lower end of the femur or the upper end of the tibia is involved).

Osteomyelitis in an older child will probably not effect the growth plate. However the blood supply to the growth plate concerned may be actually increased as a result of the infection and this may cause a stimulus of growth. Such children may in fact end up with a slightly longer limb than normal. This increase of length does not usually require treatment.

Trauma

The long bones in children unite readily. If the fracture is reduced end to end the child may finish with the limb slightly longer than it was before. The fracture of the shaft of the femur in a child reduced perfectly may result in the limb being as much as 1.5 cm longer after a year or eighteen months. If malunion is allowed to occur, however, there may well be significant shortening.

Certain fractures will damage the epiphyseal plate. Particularly important are fractures involving the lower end of the femur or the upper end of the tibia. After such fractures in the young child, a very significant shortening can develop on reaching maturity.

Neurological lesions

A paralysed limb will usually be a short limb. Leg length discrepancy occurs particularly in childen with poliomyelitis and the affected limb may be very much shorter than the other. Paraplegic children with meningomyelocele develop very short paralysed limbs. Even children with cerebral palsy are found to have the most affected limb shorter than the other.

Other causes

Arteriovenous fistulae tend to cause increase in leg length. Patients with haemangiomata may have the affected limb longer than normal or shorter than normal. Patients with neurofibromatosis may develop a gigantism of one limb or a portion of a limb.

TREATMENT OF LEG LENGTH DISCREPANCY

Less than one centimetre

Patients with such a discrepancy usually require no treatment and will not have any significant symptoms from the discrepancy.

One to three centimetres
These patients can be treated by putting a raise on the shoe of the affected side. Usually the raise on the heel is greater than that on the sole. In general terms, it is found that if the heel is restored to within 1 cm of the normal side and the sole to within 1.5 cm, an acceptable equilibrium is obtained.

Three to five centimetres
These patients can be treated by shortening the long leg. This is usually done by an operation known as an epiphysiodesis. Most of the growth in the lower limb takes place at the lower end of the femur and the upper end of the tibia. It is possible to estimate how much growth is liable to take place at these sites in any particular child. If growth is stopped at the right time, it is possible to equalise the leg lengths within a fraction of a centimetre.

Five to ten centimetres
Such a severe discrepancy is usually treated by a leg lengthening operation. This demands special apparatus. The leg is fractured subperiosteally. The apparatus is set up and the limb is gradually stretched (about one-sixteenth of an inch per day). The operation is liable to be complicated by nerve and vascular symptoms and signs in the limb. In the older child, it is usually necessary to supplement the osteotomy with a cancellous bone graft. About 10 cm in length can be obtained by this method.

Over ten centimetres
These patients nearly always require provision of an extension prosthesis and most deformities can be accommodated by one. Some children have such bizarre deformities that partial correction by surgery is required before a prosthesis can be fitted.

CHAPTER 5

Metabolic Bone Disease

Several conditions are included in this category. Osteoporosis is the most common of them and is of uncertain origin.

OSTEOPOROSIS

Osteoporosis can be defined as a condition of bone in which there is a reduction in bone mass associated with decreased production of osteoid. The chemical composition of the bone is normal. This process occurs naturally to some extent in old age. Because of this reduction in bone mass the bones become weaker and are liable to fracture (Fig. 5.1).

The causes of osteoporosis can be classified as:
1. Idiopathic (primary).
2. Disuse.
3. Due to steroid therapy (and similarly in Cushing's disease).
4. Thyrotoxicosis and acromegaly.
5. Alcoholism and liver disease.
6. Abnormal collagen metabolism – scurvy and osteogenesis imperfecta.

Idiopathic osteoporosis
This condition is very common indeed and causes considerable distress. It usually occurs in post-menopausal women. Patients complain of bone pain, particularly severe back pain. Wedging of vertebrae can cause kyphosis and loss of height (Fig. 5.2). There is a predisposition to fractures, the most common being crush fractures of the vertebral bodies, fractures of the neck of the femur and fractures of the wrist.

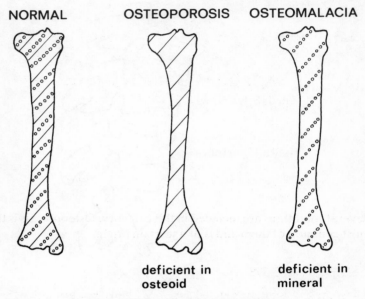

NORMAL   OSTEOPOROSIS   OSTEOMALACIA

deficient in   deficient in
osteoid   mineral

Fig. 5.1   Osteoporosis and osteomalacia.

The diagnosis is made by exclusion of other conditions with a similar presentation such as osteomalacia, secondary carcinomatosis and myelomatosis. Osteoporotic patients have no detectable biochemical abnormalities. The X-rays show a diffuse and generalised decrease in bone density. In particular, the vertebral bodies appear affected, tending to become fish-tailed in appearance with 'expansion' of the intervertebral discs. They are also inclined to fracture and become wedge-shaped as they collapse. The bone biopsy will reveal only non-specific decrease in bone mass.

Treatment of the underlying condition is unsatisfactory. Anabolic steroids, calcium supplements, vitamin D and fluoride are used but with no dramatic success.

The main complaint is of back pain. A lumbo-sacral corset may well afford relief. It is best to encourage patients to keep active and to treat them with supplements of vitamin D and calcium and advice about normal diet. Many old people living by themselves suffer from some degree of malnutrition and vitamin deficiency.

Severe incapacitating back pain associated with a crush fracture

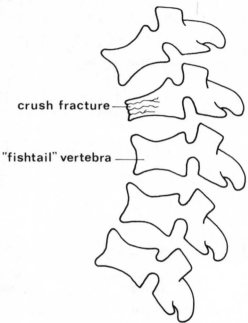

crush fracture

"fishtail" vertebra

Fig. 5.2   Osteoporosis of the spine.

can be treated with bed rest, but only for a few days. Following this, normal activity should be encouraged as soon as possible.

Fractures of the neck of the femur, of the upper end of the humerus, and Colles' fracture occur frequently in patients with osteoporosis. These tend to be more comminuted than fractures in normal bone, and more difficult to fix internally. However, the actual union of such a fracture is not a particular problem.

Disuse osteoporosis
This occurs after immobilistion as of a fractured limb in plaster. It also occurs in patients with paralysed limbs such as those with poliomyelitis or spina bifida.

After immobilisation there is a very rapid loss of bone substance. This is probably due to an alteration of the pattern of blood supply to the bone with the loss of muscle activity. It has been shown that a decrease of blood supply reduces bone formation and increases bone reabsorption.

Steroid osteoporosis
Steroid therapy is associated with a very marked and severe osteoporosis. Patients with rheumatoid arthritis who have been on steroids for any length of time develop an incapacitating osteoporosis.

OSTEOMALACIA

Osteomalacia (Fig. 5.1) can be defined as a condition in which osteoid is normally produced but mineralisation is defective. This is due to an insufficiency of available calcium or phosphate in the extracellular fluid. This picture is usually complicated by a secondary hyperparathyroidism. It is necessary to maintain blood calcium levels; parathormone will reduce calcium available for bone formation in order to maintain the blood calcium level.

Causes
   1. Dietary lack of calcium or phosphate. This is uncommon but has been described particularly when exacerbated by multiple pregnancies.
   2. Lack of vitamin D in diet. Vitamin D is necessary for the efficient assimilation of calcium from the gut.
   3. Malabsorption syndromes such as steatorrhoea which interfere with absorption both of calcium and vitamin D.
   4. Renal disease resulting in excessive loss of calcium and diminished availability of calcium.

Symptoms
   1. Bone pain, particularly in weight-bearing bones.
   2. Difficulty in walking because of pain and because of muscle weakness.
   3. Deformities, particularly kyphosis due to wedging of vertebral bodies.
   4. Specific symptoms and signs of hypocalcaemia such as paraesthesiae and spasm.

Diagnosis
   1. The alkaline phosphatase is usually raised.
   2. The serum calcium may be lowered. The urinary calcium is usually low and the faecal calcium high.
   3. X-rays show a diffuse rarefaction – some trabeculae may

appear coarse and more prominent. Areas of lysis are sometimes seen and are known as Looser's zones ('pseudo-fractures').

4. A bone biopsy will show seams of unmineralised osteoid.

The condition is treated by supplements of vitamin D and of calcium and treatment of the predisposing lesion.

RICKETS

Rickets occur in children with growing bones who have little available serum calcium and phosphate. The most marked manifestation is at the epiphyseal growth plate. The developing cartilage and newly-formed osteoid fail to calcify. The plates are therefore widened and macroscopically appear to be swollen. Growth is inhibited and the patients are stunted. Deformities occur in the weakened bones and also at the deranged growth plates. X-rays show widened epiphyseal plates and large irregular metaphyses. In addition there will be a generalised rarefaction and many deformities. Biochemistry will show a raised alkaline phosphatase and possiby a lowered serum calcium.

There are various types of rickets:

1. Dietary rickets. Caused by a diet with insufficient vitamin D.

2. Rickets due to malabsorption syndromes, such as steatorrhoea and gluten sensitivity. Calcium and vitamin D are inefficiently absorbed from the gut. Vitamin D_3 enhances calcium absorption from the gut.

3. Renal rickets (renal osteodystrophy). Patients present with chronic renal failure, stunted growth and multiple deformities. Probably calcium is unavailable because of renal loss and acidosis. The normal kidney may form the active metabolite of vitamin D_3 which actually promotes absorption of calcium from the gut.

4. Vitamin D resistant rickets (hypophosphataemia). There are several syndromes of varying severity described. The patient has a lesion of the proximal tubules of the kidney which permits loss of phosphate and various other substances.

Treatment

Treatment of rickets depends on the type of lesion. Dietary rickets can be rapidly corrected by supplements of vitamin D and calcium. That due to malabsorption syndromes requires similar treatment as well as management of the underlying condition. The bone changes of renal rickets can be considerably improved by treatment with vitamin D. Hypophosphataemic rickets require large doses of vitamin D to correct the bone changes. Surgical correction of bone deformities may be necessary.

HYPERPARATHYROIDISM

Primary hyperparathyroidism is due to excess secretion of parathormone and may be due to a parathyroid adenoma.

Most patients present with urinary symptoms due to renal calculi. The majority of these will not show any significant X-ray changes. About 15 per cent of patients present primarily with skeletal symptoms such as bone aches and pains. Some will have multiple swellings or pathological fractures. The earliest X-ray signs are seen as small erosions on the phalanges of the hands. In some cases, diffuse cystic changes are apparent (osteitis fibrosa cystica).

These patients will have a raised calcium and often a low serum phosphate (unless there is associated kidney failure). The alkaline phosphatase may be raised.

Secondary hyperparathyroidism occurs when excessive parathormone secretion is required to keep the serum calcium at its normal level. Such secondary hyperparathyroidism is seen in conditions like osteomalacia and secondary carcinomatosis. In these patients there will be diffuse thinning of bones but the more florid changes are not often seen.

VITAMIN C DEFICIENCY

Vitamin C deficiency is much less common than in earlier times. Overt scurvy in adults is very rare. However, a subclinical form of vitamin C deficiency is often present in old people in certain cities.

Patients with infantile scurvy have general symptoms of failure to thrive. In addition they show mouth haemorrhages, bone tenderness with subperiosteal haemorrhages and in due course skeletal deformities. These symptoms are probably due to the inefficient production of collagen. Vitamin C is necessary to permit the formation of hydroxyproline which is one of the amino acids specifically required in the composition of collagen protein.

CHAPTER 6

Bone Infection

ACUTE OSTEOMYELITIS

This may be a primary blood-borne infection following bacteraemia or septicaemia. It may occur, unfortunately, secondary to either trauma or surgery. Such secondary osteomyelitis is theoretically avoidable.

Acute osteomyelitis must be treated urgently and efficiently. Once infection is established in bone, it is very difficult to eradicate. If it is not eradicated, the patient will suffer a most distressing and prolonged disability.

Staphylococcus is the usual infecting organism but *Haemophilus influenzae, Salmonella* or other organisms may be responsible. It occurs commonly in children, but also occurs in adults. In neonates it has a slightly different presentation.

The commonest site for the lesion is in the metaphysis of long bones. As it is a blood-borne infection, it is potentially multifocal but usually only one site is evident.

Once established in the metaphysis the infection may spread through the adjacent cortex and form a subperiosteal abscess (Fig. 6.1a). If this occurs the blood supply to this area of cortex will be lost. The Volkmann's canals will be occluded by infection and the periosteum will be raised, interrupting the blood supply, and this area of cortex will die (Fig. 6.1b). An area of dead bone which is infected is known as a sequestrum. If this is large enough, it is almost impossible for it to be reabsorbed by normal processes, and it will form a nidus of chronic osteomyelitis (Fig. 6.1c).

The infection may also spread down the medullary cavity. The epiphyseal growth plate acts as a barrier to the spread of infection to

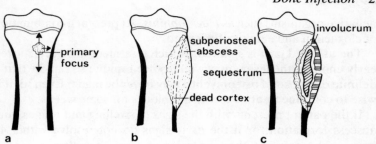

Fig. 6.1 Stages of osteomyelitis. After Crawford Adams J. (1976). *Outline of Orthopaedics*, 8th Edition. Edinburgh, Churchill Livingstone.

the adjacent joint. In neonates it is possible for infection to find its way into the joint from the metaphysis across the growth plate cartilage.

Children with osteomyelitis present with early signs and symptoms:

1. Bone pain.
2. Bone tenderness.
3. Pyrexia.

Patients with these signs may well have the lesion confined to the metaphysis, but they should be investigated and treated immediately as though they had osteomyelitis. Treatment must not wait until the diagnosis is fully confirmed.

Later signs of osteomyelitis in children are:

1. Signs of inflammation in the affected area.
2. Swelling.
3. Abscess formation.

Patients with these signs probably have a subperiosteal abscess. The adjacent area of cortex may have already become avascular and has a chance of becoming a sequestrum.

Treatment

Investigations should be started at once and should include a blood culture, an X-ray (which will probably show nothing at this stage) and a full blood count and sedimentation rate.

Antibiotics are then given, preferably intravenously. The relevant antibiotics are those that will be effective against the local *Staphylococcus* and those that will be effective against Gram-negative organisms such as *Haemophilus*. At present a combination of cloxacillin and amoxycillin is used.

The affected part is splinted. If such treatment has been started early enough, the lesion may well resolve rapidly; so rapidly that a definite diagnosis of osteomyelitis may never be made. Even so, it is wise to continue treatment with antibiotics for some weeks.

If the patient presents with the signs of swelling and redness and abscess formation, or if the early signs do not resolve within 48 hours with treatment, then the lesion requires operation.

The operation involves incision of the subperiosteal abscess. At the same time, it is wise to decompress the primary focus by removing a piece of the overlying cortex, which may in any case have lost its blood supply.

Antibiotics must be continued for a long period of time. The affected part should be immobilised until pain subsides.

In neonates, osteomyelitis presents slightly differently. The infection may spread across the epiphyseal plate into the joint and septic arthritis is more frequent. In addition, there may be permanent damage to the epiphysis. These patients also have septicaemia and are often very ill. Treatment is required to alleviate this and osteomyelitis may not be noticed until later.

Neonates

Neonates with osteomyelitis can present with a pseudo-palsy. Osteomyelitis of the upper end of the humerus in the newborn child may mimic a birth palsy.

Bone abscess (Brodie's abscess)

Patients may present with an attenuated form of osteomyelitis resulting from exposure to antibiotics for other symptoms. There will be bone pain and an X-ray will show a lesion in the metaphysis. This represents a localised abscess which requires treatment with antibiotics and surgical evacuation.

CHRONIC OSTEOMYELITIS

Chronic osteomyelitis is the sequela of inadequately treated acute osteomyelitis. There is persistent bone infection which will not be eradicated until the sequestrum is removed.

There may also be an involucrum which is formed from the raised periosteum of the subperiosteal abscess.

Treatment of chronic osteomyelitis is very difficult. It involves excising the sequestrum which may be impossible to identify. In addition, the lesion is enclosed in a mass of poorly vascularised fibrous tissue. Antibiotics are not very effective as the blood supply to the lesion is so poor. Repeated operations may be necessary and unfortunately are only partially successful. Recrudescences of the infection occur many years after the lesion has apparently resolved.

Patients with chronic osteomtyelitis have a persistent recurring disability and they may develop the following complications:

1. A persistent discharging sinus.
2. Chronic ill-health and a tendency for amyloid disease.
3. Pathological fractures and deformities.
4. Malignancy in an ulcer or in the sinus track.

SECONDARY OSTEOMYELITIS

Secondary osteomyelitis is theoretically preventible. It occurs after compound fractures and surgical operations. It should be avoided by:

1. Meticulous treatment of compound fractures.
2. Meticulous observance of septic precautions during orthopaedic operations.

Fixing fractures with metal introduces a foreign body and can lead to secondary osteomyelitis. The lesion will not resolve until all foreign material has been removed.

BONE AND JOINT TUBERCULOSIS

Tuberculosis occurs in bone and joints. The condition is still common in undeveloped countries. It also occurs in civilised western communities but not nearly so commonly as previously.

The disease is blood-borne and a focus may develop in a synovial joint or in bone. If the lesion settles in the synovium of joints it may progress gradually, producing a swollen painful joint. Gradually the joint will be destroyed.

The commonest site in bone is in the spine and the lesion is adjacent to the discs. It tends to progress on either side of the disc and eventually caseation ensues and the spine collapses into kyphotic position (Fig. 6.2). The lesions in the spine may result in paraplegia. This is probably caused by interference with the blood supply of the spinal cord as much as from the kyphus and the cold abscess.

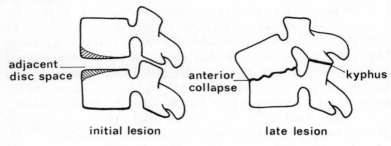

Fig. 6.2   Tuberculosis of the spine.

In early cases treatment is with antibiotics and splintage of the affected joint. It is reasonable to perform a synovectomy in early cases of joint infection. In most cases it is necessary to eradicate the infection surgically and either arthrodese or perform an excision arthroplasty of the joint. Disease of the spine is commonly treated by evacuation of the abscess and bone grafting to stabilise the spine.

CHAPTER 7

Vascular Disorders of Bone

Loss of blood supply causes local death of bone. If the lesion is very small it may be completely resolved by granulation tissue which in due course is replaced by bone. If the lesion is larger only its peripheral part can be replaced by granulation tissue. In the more central parts of the lesion, blood vessels do not develop sufficiently to support granulation tissue so the central area consists of persistent necrotic bone which is walled off by fibrous tissue. Such a large lesion heals only partially and the central infarcted portion remains.

Infarcts in subchondral bone adjacent to the joint will eventually collapse and will cause early degenerative changes to occur in that joint, as seen in Caisson disease and in sickle-cell anaemia.

Massive infarcts can occur and cause gross avascular necrosis. Such necrosis is seen particularly in the head of the femur. Collapse of such a large lesion can cause incapacitating symptoms in the hip joint.

AVASCULAR NECROSIS

This is a term used to describe infarction of a substantial portion of bone. The most frequent site is the head of the femur and the greater part of the head of the femur is involved. In due course, the infarcted area collapses and the hip joint becomes very painful (Fig. 7.1).

Avascular necrosis also occurs fairly frequently in other sites:
1. Head of the humerus.
2. Body of the talus.
3. The lunate bone (Kienbock's disease).

25

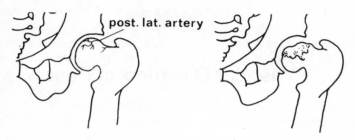

blood supply: avascular necrosis
head of femur   with collapse of head

Fig. 7.1   Avascular necrosis.

4. The condyles of the femur, producing osteonecrosis, which is seen after prolonged steroid therapy.

The commonest cause is trauma, in particular a subcapital fracture of the neck of the femur. The retinacular vessels which supply the head of the femur are frequently disrupted by the fracture.

Other causes can be listed:
1. Trauma.
   Subcapital fractures, dislocation of the hip.
   Trauma with no fracture or dislocation.
2. Slipped upper femoral epiphysis.
3. Steroid therapy.
4. Alcoholism.
5. Secondary to rheumatoid arthritis or osteoarthritis.
6. Caisson disease, sickle-cell anaemia.
7. Idiopathic.

In the early stages, the patient will complain of pain and ache in the hip which gradually become more severe. The pain may become so severe that weight bearing is intolerable.

X-ray changes do not appear until later. The affected area looks more dense and later the head will appear collapsed. The increased density may be due to micro-fractures in the infarcted area and it may also be enhanced by the rarefaction that occurs in neighbouring bone.

Treatment

In young patients, relief of weight bearing for some months may permit reconstitution. This can be accelerated by an osteotomy.

Usually, however, collapse of the head is inevitable and the hip joint must be eradicated. In older patients, a total hip replacement is the operation of choice. In young patients, arthrodesis of the hip is a rational alternative although technically difficult.

OSTEOCHONDROSIS (OSTEOCHONDRITIS)

These conditions can be described as degenerative conditions of the epiphysis which are not due to inflammation or to infection. They are probably due to repeated episodes of infarction which may be induced by trauma.

They are found in growing children. Patients complain of pain and symptoms related to a specific site. Characteristic X-ray changes are seen and the diagnosis depends on these. Usually there are no other relevant diagnostic criteria. The condition appears to be self-limiting. The lesions practically always heal but they may leave some residual deformity.

Some of the common conditions include:

1. *Perthes' disease* Occurs in the upper femoral epiphysis and is most common in boys between the ages of three and eight years.

2. *Scheurmann's disease* Occurs in the epiphyseal plates of the vertebral bodies, usually in the dorsal but also in the lumbar spine. It occurs in adolescence.

3. *Osgood-Schlatter's disease* Occurs in the tibial tuberosity of active children between the ages of seven and thirteen years.

4. *Kohler's disease* Seen in younger children and affects the navicular. Sometimes found as a chance X-ray finding and almost always heals without any significant sequelae.

OSTEOCHONDRITIS DISSECANS

This condition is found most frequently in the knee joint. The most common site is the lateral side of the medial femoral condyle (close to the attachment of the posterior cruciate ligament). It is also occasionally found in the capitellum of the elbow joint or in the talus. It consists of a localised necrotic area of bone and cartilage which is demarcated from the rest of the joint. It is probable that the area affected loses its blood supply as a result of trauma. In some patients, there is a demonstrable hereditary predisposition and, in these, more than one site may be affected. The condition is most common in 10–25 year old males.

PAGET'S DISEASE

This is a disease of the elderly (Fig. 7.2). It may involve one or many bones, of the pelvis, limbs and vertebrae; the skull is often affected.

The bones are very vascular with abnormal blood vessels. Bone is reabsorbed and laid down along these abnormal vessels and thus the internal architecture of the bone is disorganised.

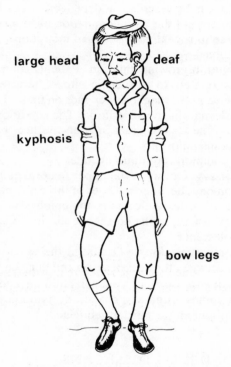

large head   deaf

kyphosis

bow legs

Fig. 7.2   Paget's disease.

Owing to the abnormal architecture the bones are weakened and become deformed; pathological fractures tend to occur. In addition, sarcomatous changes may occur producing a type of osteosarcoma. This type of osteosarcoma is practically untreatable and invariably fatal.

High output heart failure is also described as occurring in Paget's disease.

X-rays will show areas of increased density in the bones affected with alteration of the normal trabecular pattern. The bones may be expanded and deformed and pathological fractures may be seen.

The only biochemical abnormality is a raised alkaline phosphatase which can reach very high levels.

Patients may complain of deformities, such as bow legs, and of pain. This pain may arise in the bones from the disease itself, or be due to degenerative disease of joints predisposed to by bone deformities. Back pain can be caused by spinal canal stenosis, secondary to expanded vertebral bodies and pedicles. In severe cases, the skull is enlarged and thickened and the patient may have severe nerve deafness.

Treatment
Severe pain due to degenerative joint disease or vertebral stenosis can be relieved by operation. Pathological fractures are very difficult to manage and technically difficult to fix internally.

Bone pain has been treated with a variety of agents. Calcitonin is probably as effective as any, although at present it is a very expensive form of therapy.

BONE CYSTS

A cyst is defined as a collection of gas or fluid enclosed in a capsule. Haemorrhage into bone can be partially reabsorbed and cysts will result; this is seen after trauma and in patients with haemophilia. A unicameral bone cyst may result from haemorrhage into the metaphyseal region of bone.

Unicameral bone cysts
These occur in children or adolescents, who present with bone pain either from a pathological fracture or because the lesion is very near becoming a fracture. The lesion consists of a cyst which contains clear fluid and is lined by a thin layer of tissue.

The cysts usually occur in the metaphysis of long bones (the most common site is the upper end of the humerus).

Treatment
No treatment is required unless there is a fracture. If the patient is having continual pathological fractures, it is worth excising the cyst and packing the excised area with bone grafts.

Aneurysmal bone cysts
These are not common lesions. They occur in children and young people. They may present with swelling if the lesion is towards the end of long bones, or with pain from pathological fractures.

The lesion can also be found in the vertebral column and there may be symptoms of cord compression. The lesion consists of an aggregate of thin-walled, blood-filled channels, and can erode the cortex of bones. The X-ray shows an expanded lesion towards the epiphysis of a long bone (but it will not transgress the epiphyseal line unless it is closed). Aneurysmal bone cysts may be superimposed on other lesions such as osteosarcomas.

Treatment
This consists of curetting and bone graft. If the lesion is completely removed, healing will probably take place.

CHAPTER 8

Bone Tumours

The term bone tumour includes various space occupying lesions, not all of which are pathologically true tumours. Many types of primary bone tumours are rare, and on this account, diagnosis is often difficult. Only certain tumours will be considered in this section.   It must be remembered that the commonest malignant bone tumour is a secondary deposit.

CLASSIFICATION OF BONE TUMOURS

Cartilage origin

Benign
Peripheral
  Osteochondroma
Central
  Enchondroma
  Chondroblastoma
  Chondromyxoid fibroma
  Chondroid tumours

Malignant
Chondrosarcoma

Osteoblastic origin

Benign
Osteoma
Osteoid osteoma
Osteoblastoma

Malignant
Osteosarcoma
Parosteal osteosarcoma
Paget's sarcoma

Connective tissue origin

Benign
Non-osteogenic fibroma
Aneurysmal bone cyst

Malignant
Fibrosarcoma
Ewing's sarcoma

Possibly malignant
Osteoclastoma

Haematopoetic origin

Benign
Haemangioma

Malignant
Myeloma
Lymphomas
Leukaemia

Notochord origin

Malignant
Chordoma

Nerve cell origin

Benign
Neurofibroma

Fat cell origin

Benign
Lipomas

Synovial tissue origin

Malignant
Synovial sarcoma

BENIGN TUMOURS

Osteochondroma (Ecchondroma, benign exostosis)

This is a fairly common lesion (Fig. 8.1) which occurs in childhood and will slowly grow until maturity. It presents as a lump, usually on the lower end of the femur or the upper end of the tibia. The swelling is very often asymptomatic, although it occasionally may cause pressure symptoms and occasionally may fracture and become painful.

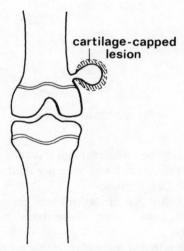

cartilage-capped
lesion

Fig. 8.1   Osteochondroma.

This lesion consists of a central core of trabecular bone covered with a cartilaginous cap. It is often in the shape of a stalk growing away from the epiphyseal plate. The active portion of the tumour is the cartilage and it may rarely progress to a chondrosarcoma. The condition of multiple osteochondromata is known as diaphysial aclasis.

X-ray shows a characteristic stalk lesion growing away from the epiphysis. If the lesion is causing symptoms, it may be excised.

Enchondroma

Enchondromata (Fig. 8.2) can be multiple, affecting the hands or the feet, and cause the condition known as enchondromatosis. The lesions are considered to arise from cartilage rests from the epiphyseal plate. These are left behind with growth in the metaphysis and proliferate to form lobular masses of cartilage which may fill the diaphysis. The patient presents with multiple swelling of hands and feet or with pathological fractures. In some patients, long bones are affected and then there may be discrepancies of leg length.

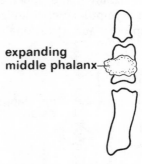

expanding
middle phalanx

Fig. 8.2   Enchondroma.

The condition may be unilateral and it is then known as Ollier's disease. It may be associated with vascular malformations, when it is known as Maffuci's syndrome.

There is a possibility that the lesions may become malignant and chondrosarcomas have been described in patients with enchondromatosis.

A solitary enchondroma can occur. If this is present in the hands or feet, it may well represent a solitary manifestation of enchondromatosis and the prognosis is similar. If it occurs more proximally in either the long bones or the bones of the pelvis or pectoral girdle, there is a greater chance of malignancy.

On X-rays, the lesion shows as a clear area of cartilage expanding the cortex. In this clear area, there may be spicules of calcification. In long bones, there is a typical streaky appearance involving the metaphysis. Enchondromata can be treated by curetting out the cartilage tumour material. If the defect is large it should be replaced with cancellous bone graft.

Osteoid osteoma

This lesion is uncommon (Fig. 8.3). Strictly it is probably not a neoplasm but, as we do not know what it is, we classify it among bone tumours. It is characterised by pain, usually well localised and becoming gradually more intense. This pain presents at night; sometimes it is relieved by aspirin.

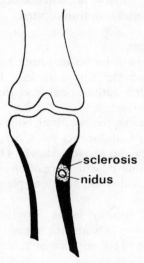

Fig. 8.3   Osteoid osteoma.

Osteoid osteoma occurs predominantly in the age group 10 – 25 and at any site. The lesion is small and therefore diagnosis is often difficult. On histology it has a particular arrangement, a central area of osteoid interspersed with vascular fibro-cellular tissue, and surrounding it an area of reactive sclerotic bone.

X-ray may show a small radiolucent nidus with a surrounding area of sclerosis. This may be difficult to interpret on plain X-rays and tomograms are invaluable in making the diagnosis.

The treatment is surgical excision which is followed by dramatic relief of symptoms. The lesion can recur if incompletely excised.

FIBROUS TISSUE LESIONS

None of these fibrous tissue lesions represent a true bone tumour. However, it is convenient to consider them here.

Fibrous cortical defect

This is a very common 'lesion' in young people. It is asymptomatic and only presents as an X-ray finding. It appears as a small lytic lesion in the cortex of long bones, usually seen in the metaphysis adjacent to the epiphyseal line. The commonest sites are the lower end of the femur and the upper end of the tibia. The defect consists of fibrous tissue and probably heals in due course.

Treatment is absolutely contraindicated.

Non-osteogenic fibroma

This is a fairly common lesion in young people, and again it is usually an asymptomatic X-ray finding. However, sometimes patients present with a pathological fracture or occasionally with pain if the cortex is infracted.

It is found in the metaphyses of long bones, usually of the lower limb. It appears as a radiolucency on X-ray, involving one cortex and adjacent medulla and expands slowly. On histology it consists of spindle cells (fibroblasts) which are often arranged in whorls and also of macrophages which contain blood pigment. Osteoid is never present.

The lesion itself usually heals spontaneously at maturity. Pathological fractures will heal with normal treatment. A painful lesion with infraction of the cortex may require curetting and bone grafting.

Fibrous dysplasia

This condition is usually seen in children and young people who may present with pathological fractures or deformities. The deformities occur when the lesion affects the bones of the skull or the face.

The lesion may be single – monostotic fibrous dysplasia – or multiple – polyostotic fibrous dysplasia. A polyostotic fibrous dysplasia may be confined to one limb and cause leg length discrepancy. Albright's syndrome is described as a polyostotic fibrous dysplasia associated with precocious puberty and areas of skin pigmentation.

The lesion consists of replacement of areas of cancellous bone (usually in the metaphysis and shafts of long bones) by primitive fibrous tissue. As the lesion progresses the fibrous tissue involves the cortex and expands it. As a result the bone is weakened and deformities and pathological fractures will result.

On histology, areas of primitive fibrous tissue are seen

interspersed with spicules of primitive bone. X-ray shows the lesion as an area of uniform density ('ground-glass appearance') which tends to scallop and expand the cortex. The bone may be expanded and bent. The lesion is usually confined to the shaft and the metaphysis of the bone. If the lesion is painful or causing a pathological fracture, it can be treated by local removal by curettage and replaced with cancellous bone graft. This can be accompanied by an osteotomy to correct deformity.

MALIGNANT BONE TUMOURS

Secondary deposits are the commonest form of malignant bone tumour. Primary malignant bone tumours are rare.

A bone tumour registry is invaluable in helping to diagnose these rare tumours. Their diagnosis depends on certain criteria.

Clinical criteria
  1. Age of the patient.
  2. The bone and the site of the bone involved.
  3. Persistent severe bone pain which may be worse at night and not relieved by rest.
  4. Swelling of the part with associated increase in temperature and dilation of overlying vessels.

X-rays
  1. A correct density properly centred X-ray of the bone involved is mandatory.
  2. Skeletal survey may be very helpful.
  3. A chest X-ray is essential.
  4. Tomograms and arteriograms are also useful.

Scan
Bone scan should be performed to show the extent of the lesion and exclude metastases. The scan may well be positive before any lesion is visible on X-ray.

Biochemistry
Investigations should include:
  1. Acid and alkaline phosphatase.
  2. Serum calcium and inorganic phosphate.
  3. Sedimentation rate and white cell count.

4. Protein electrophoresis.
5. Bone marrow smear.

Biopsy
To diagnose a primary bone tumour, an *open biopsy* is essential. This biopsy must be adequate and include some normal bone from the margin of the lesion as well as representative portions of the lesion itself.

Osteosarcoma
This is a very malignant lesion (Fig. 8.4) which occurs in young people between the ages of 10 and 30. The commonest site of the lesion is around the knee joint, the lower end of the femur and the upper end of the tibia. Patients present with symptoms of bone pain. Swelling in the region and other symptoms occur later.

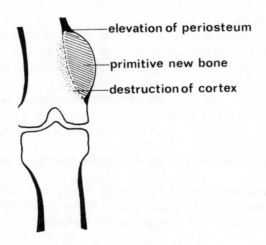

elevation of periosteum

primitive new bone

destruction of cortex

Fig. 8.4   Osteosarcoma.

The lesion is usually centrally placed and spreads along the medullary cavity and also through the cortex, eventually raising the periosteum and disrupting it, producing a soft tissue swelling. Histologically there is a very variable picture with pleomorphic sarcomatous cells which produce osteoid. There may be other tissues present as well. The lesion is very malignant and the most optimistic series only claims a 20 per cent five-year survival rate.

The X-rays show firstly a patchy destruction of the cortex at the site of the lesion. Later there is elevation of the periosteum (Codman's triangle) and finally soft tissue swelling. This may be accompanied by the so-called sunray appearance.

The treatment consists of:

1. Open biopsy.
2. Amputation covered by a combination of chemotherapeutic drugs.

This regime has in certain centres increased the overall survival rate. However there is a very high incidence of complications from the combination of chemotherapy.

Other osteosarcomas

Other types of osteosarcoma occur:

1. Paget's sarcoma occurs in older people who have Paget's disease. This is very malignant and almost uniformly fatal.
2. Parosteal osteosarcoma. This is a slow growing osteoid forming tumour which is situated in relation to the periosteum. It is less malignant than an osteosarcoma and can be treated by a wide local excision.

Chondrosarcoma

Chondrosarcomas are slow growing malignant tumours of cartilage which tend to metastasise late. The lesions are commonly proximal, in the pelvis, the bones of the pectoral girdle or in the proximal ends of long bones. They are rarely found in peripheral bones. They may arise secondary to osteochondroma or enchondroma.

The patient complains of swelling and pain. If an osteochondroma becomes painful then the diagnosis of chondrosarcoma should be considered. X-ray shows a swelling with the density of soft tissue. In this swelling areas of calcification are seen. The tumour in gross appearance appears to be lobulated and made from cartilage or it may have a gelatinous appearance.

The histology shows malignant cells which may appear like chondrocytes or chondroblasts. However there is a very variable appearance with areas of myxomatous degeneration and the lesion may be difficult to diagnose.

Treatment

Radiotherapy and chemotherapy have little effect. Radical removal of the tumour can cure the lesion. This often involves a mutilating amputation such as the hind quarter or fore quarter amputation.

In certain sites some experienced authorities have recommended a radical local excision, as the lesion is so slow growing and is so slow to metastasise.

Osteoclastoma (giant cell tumour of bone)

These lesions (Fig. 8.5) occur towards the ends of long bones in patients aged usually between 20 and 40. They are of varying malignancy. Even if the lesion is initially benign it may become malignant and cases have been described where the lesion has been irradiated and a malignant tumour has been superimposed on the benign lesion at a later date.

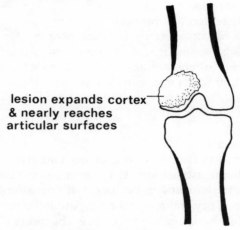

lesion expands cortex & nearly reaches articular surfaces

Fig. 8.5   Osteoclastoma.

The commonest site is around the knee, the lower end of the femur or the upper end of the tibia. The lesions also occur commonly at the wrist, in the lower end of the radius.

The X-ray appearance shows a radiolucent expanding lesion at the end of the long bone. It expands the cortex and may reach the articular surface (but rarely transgresses it). On histology the lesion is found to show giant cells and also spindle cells much like fibroblasts. The degree of malignancy is usually assessed from the study of these spindle cells.

The treatment consists of *en bloc* excision of the lesion. Following this the joint can be arthrodesed. In a convenient situation such as the knee, a custom made prosthesis can be inserted, either at the original operation or as a secondary procedure.

Myeloma
This usually presents as a multicentric tumour occurring in an older age group. It is rarely seen before the age of 40. The tumour itself is much more common than either osteosarcoma or chondrosarcoma. The patients present with bone pains or even pathological fractures. The commonest site is in the bones of the vertebral column.

Patients will also have generalised illness. Symptoms will arise from involvement of both the bone marrow, which causes anaemia and even pathological bleeding, and the kidneys. Patients often die of the kidney involvement.

Investigations
Investigations should include:

1. Blood film, which will reveal anaemia and an excess of peripheral plasma cells.

2. Blood protein, which will be raised, in particular the gammaglobulin fraction.

3. Biochemistry, possibly showing a raised serum calcium.

4. Urine, which will often reveal the presence of a Bence-Jones protein.

5. A bone marrow examination, showing excess plasma cells, often confirming the diagnosis.

6. X-ray, showing generalised osteoporosis. The typical lesions are shown as punched out areas of osteolysis. These occur particularly in the skull and in the ribs. Pathological fractures may be shown.

Treatment
This consists of cytotoxic drugs and steroids. Individual lesions may be treated by radiotherapy. If pathological fractures occur in a long bone, it should be operated on and fixed internally before radiotherapy.

Secondary metastases
Secondary metastases quite commonly form deposits in bone (Fig. 8.6). In the male the lung and the prostate are the most common primaries; in the female the breast. Carcinoma of the breast and carcinoma of the prostate have a predilection for bone. Lesions are usually multiple occurring in the vertebrae and proximal bones and also the skull and ribs.

Patients present with bone pain, which is persistent and not

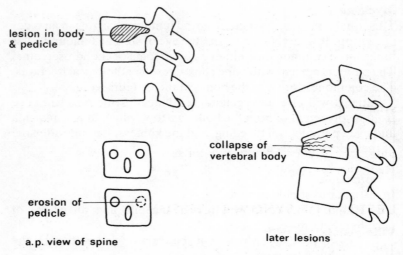

lesion in body & pedicle

collapse of vertebral body

erosion of pedicle

a.p. view of spine

later lesions

Fig. 8.6   Secondary metastases in spine.

relieved by rest, and sometimes with fractures. In the vertebrae these are crush fractures and are stable but painful. Fractures also occur in proximal long bones and will cause a considerable amount of distress unless operated and fixed internally. Secondaries occur quite commonly with carcinoma of the kidney and carcinoma of the thyroid. Symptoms from such secondaries are often the first indication of the disease.

Investigations
1. Chest X-ray.
2. Full blood count and ESR.
3. Biochemistry – calcium, phosphate, alkaline and acid phosphatase.
4. Plasma proteins.
5. Skeletal survey.
6. Bone scan.
7. Bone marrow.
8. Bone biopsy. With secondaries it is permissible to use a needle biopsy rather than open operation.

If the patient presents with a secondary deposit then a full-scale search must be made to find the primary cause of the lesion. The X-ray appearances of the lesion may reveal a pathological fracture.

The lesions are usually osteolytic with a diffuse margin and they rarely cause expansion of the involved bone. Carcinoma of the prostate are classically osteoblastic.

Treatment
Treatment of the primary tumour may relieve the patient's symptoms significantly. Cytotoxic drugs have an important part to play in the treatment of metastatic carcinoma. Radiotherapy may be used for a specific lesion. If a pathological fracture occurs in a long bone it is mandatory to operate on it and fix it internally. Radiotherapy may then be given.

LESIONS OF SYNOVIAL TISSUE

Villo-nodular synovitis
This condition probably represents a chronic inflammatory response of synovial tissue. However, it mimics a tumour and unfortunately has often been treated as such.

It occurs in adult life and is seen most commonly in the flexor tendon sheaths of the hands or feet where it presents as a nodule. It tends to proliferate between the tendons and even into the underlying bone eroding it. It is also seen in the knee joint (and other joints) where it causes a proliferative villous reaction of the synovium, which is stained brown with haemosiderin pigment. These patients complain of swelling and recurrent knee effusions.

Histology of the lesions show spindle and polyhedral cells with synovial clefts; there are also giant cells with haemosiderin pigment. In some patients the lesion appears so cellular that it can mimic a sarcoma. X-ray may show erosions of the cortex. An extensive chronic lesion can become calcified.

Patients with nodules in the flexor tendons can have these excised. This should be done meticulously as the lesion can recur from the proliferations left behind.

Synovial sarcoma
This is a malignant tumour of synovial tissue. It occurs usually in young adult life, most frequently about the knee joint.

It frequently presents as a nodule in the soft tissues about the joint and as such may be diagnosed as a meniscus cyst, ganglion or 'fibroma'. On excision however, it has a whitish-grey fleshy appearance with a false capsule. In due course, the lesion will grow and spread to become a diffuse firm swelling. Metastases occur frequently in the lungs.

On histology the lesion has sarcomatous fusiform cells with synovial clefts between them. Sometimes these cells have a 'glandular' arrangement. Treatment involves either extensive excision of the lesion followed by radiotherapy, or amputation.

CHAPTER 9

Bone Dysplasias

A dysplasia may be defined as an abnormal development of tissue.

Dysplasias of bone result from the faulty maturation of the cells involved in developing bone: fibroblasts, chondroblasts and osteoblasts. This faulty maturation may have a definite biochemical basis (as has been demonstrated in the group of conditions known as mucopolysaccharoidoses). In many conditions, other tissues besides bone are affected. Dysplasias often have a hereditary basis.

A great many syndromes are described.

There is a wide spectrum of severity seen in patients suffering the lesions of these syndromes. An individual case may well be 'atypical'.

Clinically, patients with bone dysplasia may present in various ways:

1. In some patients the disease is so severe that it is incompatible with life, as with the most severe form of osteogenesis imperfecta.

2. Patients frequently present as dwarfs. 'Circus dwarfs' are often achondroplastics.

3. They have numerous deformities due to the abnormal shape of bones, resulting in bow legs or coxa vara, joint deformities and contractures similar to club feet.

4. They frequently have leg length discrepancy.

5. Pathological fractures may occur in these patients, particularly in those with osteogenesis imperfecta.

6. Some patients have associated systemic abnormalities affecting the skin, the heart, the brain and other systems.

7. Some of the syndromes show classical skull or facial abnormalities. The particular facial appearance of these children may be helpful in making the diagnosis.

45

8. Because of abnormalities of bone and joint shape, these patients will often develop early degenerative changes in their joints. In some cases, these patients will have symptoms severe enough to warrant treatment directed towards these degenerative changes.

CLASSIFICATION

This classification is adapted from Aegerter and Kirkpatrick.
1. Dysplasias due to abnormal cartilage growth and metabolism.
    a. Abnormal proliferation of growth plate chondroblasts, e.g. enchondromatosis or osteochondromatosis.
    b. Abnormal maturation of growth plate chondroblasts, e.g. achondroplasia or diastrophic dwarfs.
    c. Biochemical abnormalities, e.g. mucopolysaccharoidoses.

2. Dysplasias due to abnormal bone growth and metabolism.
    a. Abnormal epiphyseal centres, e.g. multiple epiphyseal dysplasia.
    b. Deficient osteoid production, e.g. osteogenesis imperfecta.
    c. Excess osteoid production, e.g. osteopetrosis, diaphyseal sclerosis.
    d. Abnormal osteoid production, e.g. fibrous dysplasia, neurofibromatosis.

3. Miscellaneous dysplasias, e.g. Marfan's syndrome, Apert's syndrome.

ACHONDROPLASIA

These patients present as dwarfs (Fig. 9.1). A great many are still-born or die as neonates; however, those who do survive have normal intelligence and may be fertile.

Many of them are of autosomal dominant inheritance but many are the outcome of mutations.

Biopsies of epiphyseal growth plates have shown a paucity and abnormal maturation of chondroblasts. The growth of bones formed in cartilage is severely affected.

The long bones of the limbs are short. The hands are broad and the fingers short. The bones of the skull base are affected so that the nose and lower part of the face appear small and the vault of the

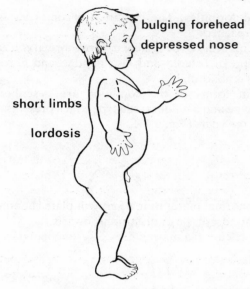

Fig. 9.1 Achondroplasia.

skull is protruberant. The foramen magnum is small and the first and second cervical vertebrae are often abnormal.

The trunk is almost of normal length but individual vertebrae have short pedicles and achondroplastics are liable to develop symptoms from vertebral stenosis in later life. They tend to have a lumbar lordosis and the sacrum may lie transversely.

X-rays show the pelvis to be small with 'spade-like' ilia. The long bones are short with flared epiphyses; the ribs are short and flat.

These people can exist independently and earn a living; some of them make use of their deformity to work as 'circus dwarfs'. They rarely present for treatment unless they develop the signs and symptoms of vertebral stenosis in later life.

OSTEOGENESIS IMPERFECTA

These patients present with multiple fractures caused by only minor trauma. There are various grades of severity. Some very severely affected are still-born; others have gross multiple fractures and deformities and will die in infancy. Other children only have an increased liability to fractures and may well be left with no significant deformities. The condition becomes less severe once adult life is reached.

The patients seem to be unable to form normal collagen and thus the formation of osteoid and also dentine and fibrous tissue in certain sites is abnormal.

Two main forms of the condition are described, a severe congenital type and a milder tarda type which presents after the age of two or three years (Fig. 9.2).

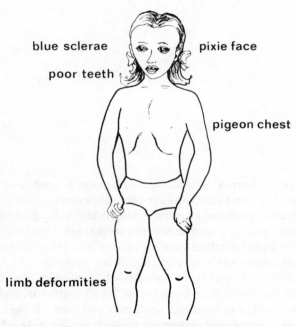

blue sclerae   pixie face

poor teeth

pigeon chest

limb deformities

Fig. 9.2   Osteogenesis imperfecta.

The severe congenital type presents with gross deformities. The patient is dwarfed. The head is large, the face small and the teeth abnormal. X-rays show grossly deformed long bones with a marked degree of osteoporosis. This type most often occurs as a spontaneous mutation.

The tarda type of patient presents with frequent fractures from minor trauma. They have a small triangular face with a broad forehead (the 'pixie face'). Patients frequently have blue sclerotics and they may develop other abnormalities such as pes excavatum and scoliosis. In later life they may become deaf.

Treatment consists of the management of fractures as they occur; union is usually uneventful. However, sometimes a grossly proliferative callus is seen which may mimic an osteosarcoma. Patients with limb deformities can have these corrected by multiple osteotomies and rodding. Various medical treatments have been tried but none have been proved to be effective.

NEUROFIBROMATOSIS

This condition is inherited as an autosomal dominant and has a variable presentation.

All patients have pigmented areas known as cafe-au-lait spots. As these are so common in normal people, it has been suggested that six or more cafe-au-lait spots over 1.5 cm in diameter are necessary to make the diagnosis.

The neurofibromata are tumours of the Schwann cells or the fibrous and supporting tissue of nerves. They are found in the skin and along nerve trunks. There is a great variation in the number and size of neurofibromata present in each patient. They can cause gross cosmetic deformities.

The tumours contain masses of spindle cells like fibroblasts. About 10 per cent will become malignant and cause pressure symptoms. The tumours will also cause symptoms if they grow in a confined space such as the spinal canal.

Neurofibromatosis is associated with a variety of skeletal abnormalities.

1. It is a cause of leg length discrepancy. There may be overgrowth of the affected limb.

2. Local gigantism of one or two digits may be seen which can be severe enough to produce a grotesque deformity.

3. Areas of demineralisation of bone are seen. The bone is replaced by neurofibromatosis tissue.

4. A particular lesion known as pseudarthrosis of the tibia is described and about 50 per cent of cases are associated with neurofibromatosis. In this condition, there is a malformation of the distal tibia which permits bowing and eventually disruption of the tibia. The condition is very resistant to grafting or any other form of therapy and the majority of patients benefit from an amputation.

5. Scalloping of vertebrae may be seen and this is associated with

abnormalities of the meninges. These abnormalities are reflected in meningoceles as seen on the myelogram.

6: Scoliosis is frequent in patients with neurofibromatosis and is difficult to treat.

CHAPTER 10

Synovial Joints

A synovial joint consists of two bearing surfaces lined by articular cartilage bonded to subchondral bone. The 'cavity' contains synovial fluid and is lined by a synovial membrane. The whole is invested by a capsule and constrained by ligaments. Some joints include menisci and fat pads (Fig. 10.1).

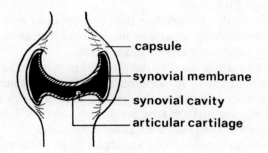

Fig. 10.1   Synovial joint.

Adult hyaline cartilage contains chondrocytes which maintain a diffuse matrix. This consists of a feltwork of collagen fibres supporting a protein polysaccharide gel. This has the property of binding water. The hyaline cartilage is firmly attached to the underlying subchondral bone by arcades of collagen fibres.

The following functions of articular cartilage should be remembered:

1. It receives nutrients from the synovial fluid.

51

2. The synovial fluid is squeezed in and out of the 'cartilage sponge' by pressure of joint movement. Such movement is necessary for the adequate maintainence of articular cartilage.

3. The cartilage is compliant and will alter shape with pressure. Thus with varying loads there is a varying area of cartilage in contact with the opposite bearing surface.

4. Cartilage has a limited capacity for repair. This is greater towards the periphery of the joint surface near the perichondrium. It is also greater if the underlying bone is involved. Primary repair is by fibroblasts to fibrocartilage; this may later metaphase to hyaline cartilage.

The backing of the joint lining consists of a layer of calcified cartilage overlying a layer of subchondral bone. Beneath this are arcades of trabecular bone (of the expanding metaphysis) which gradually give way to the normal compact tubular cortex (of the diaphysis) (see Fig. 1.4, p. 4). Note that:

1. This layer of trabecular bone gives firm support to the articular cartilage.

2. It is vascular and has a greater capacity for repair and remodelling of the joint.

3. It has greater compliance than cortical bone and its arcades will therefore cushion impacts on the joint before transmitting them to the more rigid cortical bone of the shaft.

Synovial fluid is formed by the synovial membrane as a dialysate of extracellular fluid. In addition it contains a hyaluronic acid-containing mucoprotein. In the normal adult it forms a very thin layer between the surfaces (the 'joint space' seen on X-ray is mostly cartilage space). Synovial fluid has three functions:

1. It contains nutrients for articular cartilage and is squeezed into it during joint motion.

2. It acts as a lubricant and is found to have a variable viscosity. At high rates of motion the hyaluronate molecules probably align themselves so that the viscosity of synovial fluid is lowered.

3. Human joint surfaces are slightly asymmetrical; it is possible that synovial fluid forms a wedge of lubrication. The formation of this wedge would be assisted by menisci and fat pads.

The synovial membrane lines areas of the joint which are not involved in weight bearing. It is vascular and has a nerve supply.

1. It forms synovial fluid.

2. Its cells have a phagocytic function and will remove debris from the joint.

3. Joint pain sensation is probably transmitted from the nerve endings in the synovium when it is distended.

The fibrous capsule envelopes the joint but is arranged so that it permits movement.

The ligaments are so arranged as to control joint movement along certain planes. Both capsule and ligaments have a copious nerve supply and contain proprioceptive endings. They also supply information as to joint position. By various reflex arcs, they can inhibit excessive movement which can cause damage to the joint. Patients with neurological signs associated with loss of proprioception are liable to develop florid degenerative joint disease, the so-called Charcot's joint.

Human joints are designed to permit movement between bones. They are also designed so that in a certain position the joint can be rigidly stabilised and the component bones act as a rigid pillar.

In order to permit the greatest freedom of movement:

1. The joint surfaces are usually slightly asymmetrical (to permit 'spins' as well as rolls and slides).

2. The ligaments are not always taut.

3. The capsule is lax.

CHAPTER 11

Arthritis

Arthritis is a non-specific term used to describe a pathological structural alteration of a joint.

The various types of arthritis may be classified as:

1. Degenerative disease (osteoarthritis).
2. Arthritis due to hypersensitivity reactions (rheumatoid arthritis, ankylosing spondylitis).
3. Infective arthritis.
4. Secondary arthritis (gout, haemophilia).
5. Traumatic arthritis (occurring in a joint so badly damaged that recovery is impossible).

DEGENERATIVE DISEASE (osteoarthritis)

This is a disease of people of mature years. The symptoms develop mainly in weight-bearing joints. Sufferers complain of pain on activity and loss of motion of the joint affected.

Pathology
The initial lesion appears to be atrophy of the hyaline cartilage with death of chondrocytes. Associated with this may be thickening of the synovium and decreased vascularity.

A later stage consists of 'peripheral repair' with new cartilage forming at the periphery which in due course will form new bone. Osteophytes are formed which tend to stabilize the joint and make it more symmetrical. As the cartilage disappears the underlying bone becomes more sclerosed and eburnated.

The X-ray shows a loss of joint space (loss of cartilage space). Osteophytes are seen and also 'cyst' formation.

Degenerative disease can be classified as either primary (idiopathic) or secondary to some other lesion.

Predisposing factors causing osteoarthritis are:

1. Ageing. In old people there is a diminished reparative capacity, and the blood supply to the joint may be diminished.

2. Obesity. This has an effect which is simply mechanical and also obese patients have various other lesions which may produce degenerative changes.

3. Loss of concentricity, e.g. Perthes' disease or slipped epiphysis, loose fragments such as those of meniscus or of loose bodies, trauma.

4. Malalignment. Osteoarthritis of the knee is predisposed to by bow legs or knock knees. Malunited fracture of the tibia will tend to predispose to osteoarthritis of the ankle joint.

5. Instability. Knee ligament instability will predispose to degenerative change. Congenital dislocation of the hip with the hip remaining subluxed will predispose to degenerative change.

6. Alterations in synovial fluid. This will affect the nutrition of the articular cartilage and cause degenerative changes. Such alterations occur in septic arthritis, rheumatoid arthritis, haemophilia.

7. Alteration in subchondral bone, e.g. avascular necrosis, metal implants. It is the 'backing' of the joint which is primarily affected in avascular necrosis. The 'backing' is also made more rigid by metal implants.

The symptoms of degenerative disease are more severe if the lesion is in a weight-bearing joint. In the upper limb, quite severe change may not cause significant symptoms.

The symptoms of degenerative disease are characterised by exacerbations and remissions even though the lesion itself is essentially structural. The patient can develop significant degenerative changes in their joints and complain of minimal symptoms for years. Exacerbation symptoms are liable to develop from minor trauma or from excessive use. The symptoms can often be relieved by conservative measures such as drugs, rest, temporary splintage, or some sort of physiotherapy. Many patients with degenerative disease in their joints require no more treatment than this. If their symptoms are persistent in spite of such conservative therapy then a variety of operations can be considered.

RHEUMATOID ARTHRITIS

This is a very common disease, affecting women more commonly than men. It may occur at practically any age. When it occurs in children it is known as Still's disease. Initially it may affect only one joint but in due course several joints will be involved. The commonest site is in the joints of the hands or the feet.

It is a generalised systemic disease of collagen tissue affecting other tissues besides joints. The patients are often 'ill'.

It is characterised by exacerbations and remissions, and the course is unpredictable:

1. The condition may resolve entirely.
2. The patient may suffer repeated exacerbations and remissions and be left with some degree of permanent disability.
3. It may proceed inexorably to severe disability and crippling.

The rheumatoid factor is present and identifiable in 75 per cent of those patients with *established* disease. This is probably an antibody which is stimulated by a specific antigenic gamma globulin from lymphocytes. Why this specific antigenic gamma globulin is produced is not known. It is suggested that this antibody – antigen complex is phagocytosed on the surface of synovial cells and the breakdown products cause inflammatory reaction.

The initial lesion is an inflammation of the synovium (and possibly of the subchondral bone). Other connective tissue may be involved such as the synovium of tendons. The synovium becomes thickened and undergoes hyperplasia and is filled with aggregates of lymphocytes. Exudate occurs into the joint producing an effusion. In due course this effusion is precipitated as a layer of fibrin over the articular surface (Fig. 11.1).

In the next stage granulation tissue organises the fibrin over the articular surface and forms a pannus which tends to erode the articular cartilage. A similar process occurs in the subchondral bone below the articular cartilage, in the attachments of the capsule of the joint and in the attachment of the constraining ligaments. A similar pannus is found in the synovial sheath of tendons; it may erode them and cause them to rupture (see Fig. 15.13, p. 121).

In later stages adhesions will form in the joint; these may coalesce and a fibrous ankylosis result. Secondary osteoarthritic changes may supervene on the damaged articular cartilage. If the capsule and the ligaments have been badly damaged or stretched, joint deformities or instability will result.

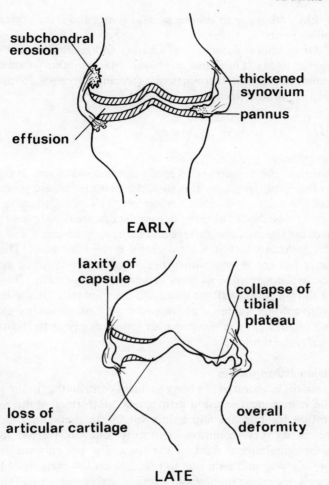

subchondral
erosion

thickened
synovium

pannus

effusion

EARLY

laxity of
capsule

collapse of
tibial
plateau

loss of
articular cartilage

overall
deformity

LATE

Fig. 11.1 Rheumatoid knee.

Treatment

These patients are best managed by a rheumatologist in co-operation with an orthopaedic surgeon.

Conservative treatment includes:

1. Bed rest in the early stages when the patient is tired and ill.

2. Splintage to relieve the pain of affected joints, to prevent contractures and to support unstable joints.

3. Physiotherapy to relieve painful joints and later exercises to mobilise joints.

4. Drug therapy including aspirin, indomethacin and other analgesic drugs. Gold has a proven place in the treatment of rheumatoid arthritis. Intra-articular steroids can be used to produce a chemical synovectomy.

SURGICAL PROCEDURES

Synovectomy

This means the excision of as much diseased synovium as possible from the joint. In theory this should arrest the disease process. In practice it may do and very frequently relieves distressing pain. Synovectomy should be done before the disease progresses too far, destroying the articular surface and damaging the capsule.

The joint in which it is most useful is the knee joint. The most suitable patient is one with a persistent boggy synovial swelling which will not resolve with conservative management. The X-ray must show a good cartilage space and the joint must be stable.

Synovectomy is often used with other procedures such as excision of the ulnar styloid combined with synovectomy of the wrist joint and extensor tendons.

Excision arthroplasties

This means excision of the bony surfaces contributing to the joint.

The commonest excision arthroplasty performed is the Keller's operation for bunions and hallux valgus. In rheumatoid arthritis there is a very common deformity due to disease of the metatarsophalangeal joint of the toes. The patients suffer from severe clawing and pain due to pressure on the metatarsal heads. Fowler's operation involves an excision arthroplasty of all the toes of the foot excising the metatarsal heads and bases of the proximal phalanges so that the toes will conform to a reasonable shape.

Arthrodesis

This means that the articular surfaces of the joint are excised and the underlying cancellous bone ends are fixed together so that the joint is obliterated. In due course the joint will be fused by bone.

In rheumatoid patients it must be remembered that rheumatoid arthritis affects many joints and that each one arthrodesed throws more strain on neighbouring joints.

Arthrodesis is the treatment of choice for rheumatoid patients with:
1. Disease of the subtalar joint.
2. Instability of the cervical spine.
3. Painful disease of the distal interphalangeal joint.

It is often useful to stabilise the thumb in rheumatoid arthritis. Arthrodeses of the wrist and knee are frequently performed.

Prosthetic joint replacement
Prosthetic joint replacements are performed frequently in patients with rheumatoid arthritis; of proven value are:
1. Total hip replacement.
2. Total knee replacement.
3. Silastic replacements of metacarpophalangeal joints of the hands.

It must be remembered that patients with rheumatoid arthritis are particularly liable to poor wound healing and post-operative infection. Stringent precautions have to be taken before inserting prosthetic replacements into these patients.

Various other procedures are performed on rheumatoid arthritic patients including release of contractures, tendon transfer, carpal tunnel decompression and removal of nodules.

SEPTIC ARTHRITIS

This condition results from infection of the joint with micro-organisms. The commonest infecting organism is *Staphylococcus*, although *Streptococcus* and *Haemophilus* are frequently involved and numerous other pathogens have also been described.

Infection may occur via the blood stream from a focus elsewhere, or it may occur secondary to trauma or a surgical operation. It can occur secondary to a focus of osteomyelitis if the metaphysis is intracapsular. Septic arthritis of the hip is often secondary to osteomyelitis in the neck of the femur (Fig. 11.2).

If the lesion is untreated the joint will become swollen and distended with fluid and later with pus. In due course the articular cartilage becomes eroded and eventually completely destroyed. Adhesions form in the joint and these later become organised to fibrous tissue. Finally a fibrous or even a bony ankylosis occurs.

Patients are usually children or young adults who present with pyrexia and an exquisitely tender and swollen joint. X-ray may

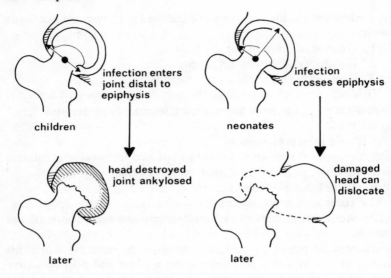

Fig. 11.2   Septic arthritis of hip.

confirm the distension but show nothing more specific in the early stages. A full blood count will reveal a leucocytosis. A blood culture may be positive for the affecting organism.

Treatment
The diagnosis can be confirmed by aspiration, usually under a general anaesthetic. The limb is splinted and antibiotics are given. Cloxacillin and amoxycillin are a good combination initially; when the organism is positively identified, the most effective antibiotics are continued for at least six weeks.

It is sometimes necessary to open the joint to decompress it and wash it out. This is usually necessary with infections of the hip joint.

If treatment is undertaken early and efficiently, the condition will resolve without serious sequelae.

Neonates are particularly difficult to diagnose as having septic arthritis. The condition usually follows a general severe infection resulting in a septicaemia and patients are therefore desperately ill. It may only be manifest by an absence of movement in a limb in a child who has been seriously ill ('pseudo-paralysis').

Septic arthritis also occurs in very old patients and in patients who have rheumatoid arthritis as a low grade condition. They may present with a warm swollen joint which is sometimes not particularly painful. Aspiration of this joint will reveal the diagnosis.

GOUT

Patients with gout are liable to recurrent attacks of arthritis. The condition is due to an abnormality of purine metabolism which results in a raised serum uric acid. They have episodes of severe arthritic pain which are associated with a raised serum uric acid (over 7.0 mg per cent). These episodes are associated with deposition of sodium biurate crystals in the affected joints.

The patients are usually males approaching middle age. They suffer recurrent attacks of severely painful arthritis. These occur initially in the metatarsophalangeal joint of the great toe, but other joints may be affected. Attacks can be precipitated by injury or operation.

In patients with long-standing disease, the affected joints tend to become disorganised. X-rays will show erosions adjacent to the joint and narrowing of the articular cartilage. In addition, deposits occur elsewhere such as the olecranon bursa and the ear lobes, forming tophi.

Treatment
Treatment is essentially medical. Phenylbutazone is most effective for acute attacks. Allopurinol reduces the formation of uric acid and is used as a long term prophylactic.

If an operation is considered for a known gout-sufferer, it is wise to 'cover' the procedure with phenylbutazone.

There are certain patients who appear to suffer a subclinical form of gout. These patients suffer excessively from minor injury to connective tissue such as rotator cuff lesions, tennis elbow and tenosynovitis. A random serum uric acid may be raised. Such patients may be considered to have a gouty diathesis and such episodes should be treated sympatheticlly but with prolonged conservative treatment.

CRYSTAL SYNOVITIS (PSEUDO-GOUT)

There are patients who develop symptoms of an acute arthritis simulating a septic arthritis. The knee joint is most commonly affected. The joint aspirate will show turbid fluid which if examined microscopically by polarised light will reveal monorefringent crystals of calcium pyrophosphate.

Sometimes there is sufficient deposition of this substance to outline the menisci (and articular surfaces) on X-ray.

Treatment is to aspirate the effusion and rest the inflamed joint. Phenylbutazone or indomethacin will rapidly relieve the symptoms.

HAEMOPHILIA

These patients (nearly always male) are subject to recurrent episodes of spontaneous bleeding, due to low levels of antihaemophilic globulin. This bleeding can occur into joints and muscles causing an acute and sometimes a chronic orthopaedic problem.

Any large joint may be involved. Bleeding will cause a painful haemarthrosis which will eventually resolve. However, repeated episodes of bleeding will cause the synovial membrane to become thickened and eventually fibrosed. In due course the articular cartilage becomes eroded and the joint becomes irreversibly damaged. Finally a fibrous ankylosis results.

The muscle group most commonly involved is the ilio-psoas. Unless the bleeding is rapidly arrested the muscle will be disorganised by haematoma and eventually a fibrous contracture will result.

Patients with joint lesions present with a warm painful swollen joint which may simulate a septic arthritis. Patients with a muscle haematoma will have a painful contracture.

Treatment

Antihaemophilic factor is now available as cryoprecipitate. This should be given intravenously and the affected joint immobilised. A patient with an ilio-psoas contracture requires skin traction to the affected limb.

If the haemarthrosis does not rapidly resolve, it should be aspirated. Fortunately the cryoprecipitate has such dramatic effect that this is not often necessary.

Patients with chronic joint disorganisation may require supportive orthoses. It is now possible to operate on badly damaged joints using cryoprecipitate 'cover' and perform a synovectomy, arthrodesis, or even a joint replacement.

NEUROPATHIC JOINTS (CHARCOT'S JOINTS)

Joints have an abundance of nerve endings situated in the synovium and capsule and adjacent ligaments. These nerve endings subserve pain and proprioception (position sense). They are involved not only with promoting normal balance and joint function, but also protect the joint. If this function is lost, the joint is liable to damage.

Classically, patients with secondary syphilis (tabes dorsalis) were found to have swollen unstable joints with florid degenerative changes. There was marked osteophyte proliferation. In spite of these severe changes, these joints were not excessively painful. These joints are now most often seen in patients with diabetes but may be found in other conditions in association with a sensory neuropathy or with lesions of the posterior columns of the spinal cord.

Treatment is difficult, and appropriate orthoses may be of value. Operative treatment is often unsatisfactory; an arthrodesis is difficult to obtain and a prosthetic replacement has a tendency to dislocate.

CHAPTER 12

Soft Tissue Lesions

TENDON LACERATIONS

When a tendon is cut the two ends retract. In order for healing to occur the severed endings must be in apposition. The area of the laceration is then surrounded by a blood clot which will organise. The organising tissue contains fibroblasts, derived from the paratenon, which will gradually form new collagen to fuse with that in the remaining ends of the tendon. A mass of 'tendon callus' results. The tendon will remodel when activity is resumed.

The majority of tendon lacerations will heal provided the two ends are adequately apposed.

Extensor tendons
The extensor tendons of the hand are frequently lacerated.

Treatment
1. The wound is explored under a tourniquet with the patient anaesthetised.
2. The tendon ends are sutured. This repair should be as meticulous as possible using non-absorbable sutures.
3. The finger is then splinted in a relaxed position for two or three weeks.
4. Graduated exercises are required as remodelling of the tendon and resolution of stiffness occurs.

Flexor tendons
If the tendon is in a sheath, the repair is more complicated. It is particularly complicated in the case of flexor tendons of the hand. The profundus and sublimis flexor tendons of the finger are in the

same synovial sheath, which extends from the distal skin crease of the palm to the distal skin crease of the finger (Fig. 12.1). In this region, the primitive cells migrate not only from the paratenon of both profundus and sublimis tendons, but also from the overlying sheath and a mass of granulation tissue can result. Normal function is unlikely to occur with resolution of this mass. Results of primary exploration and suture in this area are poor unless very special precautions are taken.

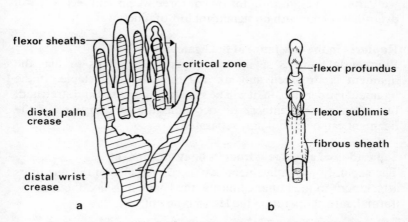

Fig. 12.1 (a) Flexor sheaths of fingers, (b) tendon insertion.

Treatment

If the wound is clean and the laceration is clear cut it is possible with the aid of an operating microscope to perform a primary repair of one or even both tendons using very fine sutures. With many patients, unfortunately, either the facilities are not available or the wound is unsuitable. It is then necessary to repair the tendon in stages:

1. Debridement of the wound with skin closure only, followed by physiotherapy to keep the finger mobile.

2. Replacement of the flexor tendons by a graft, usually from the palmaris longus.

This operation is technically difficult and the results are frequently unsatisfactory.

LIGAMENT INJURIES

If a joint is subjected to excessive violence, its collateral ligaments can be disrupted. Various grades of ligament injury occur.

Ligament sprain

If the violence is not severe enough to cause a complete disruption it can stretch or partially disrupt the ligament. This is known clinically as a 'ligament sprain'. On careful clinical examination, no laxity of the ligament can be detected. A ligament sprain can heal reasonably well after immobilisation for two or three weeks and recovery will eventually occur with no significant loss of function.

Ruptures in the substance of the ligament

Frequently there is separation of individual fibres so that the ligament is stretched and lax and the joint is unstable. If the ligament is operated on, it will be seen to be contused and stretched, but often grossly 'intact'; on occasions the two portions of the ligament can be completely separated.

Separation of a ligament from its bony attachment

The separation of a ligament may occur actually on the line of its attachment to the bone. Clinically the ligament is lax, the X-ray is normal, and at operation the lesion is obvious.

Avulsion fractures

The violence acting on the ligament can cause a fracture at its attachment to bone, pulling away a small fragment. This will be visible on X-ray. Clinically the ligament will be lax and functionless. Such avulsion fracture fragments will heal if they are accurately replaced. They may necessitate an open operation (Fig. 12.2).

Treatment

Ligament ruptures may be difficult to diagnose. If the diagnosis is suspected, it is quite reasonable to examine the joint under an anaesthetic to demonstrate the lesion. In most situations, it is adequate to splint the joint for some weeks to permit healing of the ligament.

Better results are obtained by open operation and primary repair of knee ligament injuries in young and athletic people. Such repairs must be followed by splinting for some weeks to promote

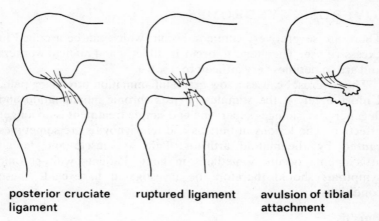

posterior cruciate   ruptured ligament   avulsion of tibial
ligament   attachment

Fig. 12.2   Rupture of posterior cruciate ligament.,

healing and thereafter graduated exercises are required to restore movement.

Chronic laxity of ligaments may be treated conservatively either by training muscles to supplement ligament function or by providing an orthosis. Some patients require operative treatment. This may involve simply reefing the lax ligament. However, it is usually necessary to supplement the ligament by re-routing an adjacent tendon. The semitendinosus muscle is frequently used for knee ligament repairs.

Ligaments not only constrain the joint and prevent subluxation through their innate strength, but also are copiously supplied with proprioceptive nerve endings. These protect the joint (and the ligaments) by initiating protective muscle activity to counteract excessive stress. When a ligament is damaged it may appear to heal satisfactorily, but it is possible that its protective proprioceptive nerve supply will not be fully restored. Operations which reconstitute ligaments with fascial strips and tendon transfers may well restore the fibrous component of the ligament but patients should be advised that the proprioceptive function may not return.

Artificial ligaments have been tried but so far have been unsuccessful. Such ligaments of course will have no proprioceptive nerve supply. Furthermore, they have no built-in repair process against fatigue failure as does living connective tissue.

'OVERUSE' SYNDROMES

There are several very common lesions which can be ascribed to excessive use. They tend to occur in athletes and manual workers and are sometimes very difficult to resolve.

The 'overuse' causes a low grade inflammation producing pain. Unfortunately if the stimulus persists chronic inflammation and degenerative changes supervene and simple treatment is no longer effective. The lesions of bursitis and tenosynovitis are sometimes caused by rheumatoid arthritis. Pain at muscle and fascial attachments occurs sometimes in gout. Patients with chronic symptoms should therefore be investigated to exclude these conditions.

Bursitis

This occurs frequently in relation to bony prominences; common types are pre-patella bursitis (housemaid's knee) and olecranon bursitis (student's elbow). Patients complain of a swelling which may be painful. Treatment involves cessation of the offending activity and the application of a pressure bandage. Occasionally aspiration and instillation of steroid is necessary.

If the lesion has become chronic, operative treatment may be helpful.

Tenosynovitis

This arises in the synovial sheaths around tendons. The patients present with pain and swelling after excessive activity. Common sites include the extensor tendons over the dorsum of the wrist and the tendo achillas 'bursa'.

Lesions of muscle and fascial attachments

In certain areas the attachment of muscles and/or of fascia is particularly liable to excessive and repeated stress. Common sites include the lateral epicondyle of elbow (tennis elbow, see Fig. 16.4, p. 127) and the posterior tubercle of calcaneus (plantar fasciitis).

Patients complain of persistent pain at the site which is worse on certain activities.

DEGENERATIVE SOFT TISSUE LESIONS

The strength of fibrous tissue is due to its constituent collagen fibres. These are embedded in a water-containing protein polysaccharide matrix. Tendons have a blood supply which supplies nutrients to the fibrocytes and these maintain collagen. With age, changes occur in tendons and ligaments;

The collagen develops more and more stable cross-linkages.

The water content of the matrix decreases and the polysaccharides tend to alter.

It is suggested that, on both these counts, it is more difficult for the fibrocytes to maintain collagen and therefore it is liable to undergo degeneration. The blood supply to the tendon may be deficient. This has been demonstrated in the tendons around the rotator cuff of the shoulder.

Degenerative changes may result in overt abnormalities:

Susceptibility to minor trauma.

The presence of areas of calcification.

A tendency to spontaneus rupture associated with imperfect and delayed healing. Such ruptures are often incomplete.

Examples of such degenerative lesions include:

Rupture of the tendo achilles (p. 250).

Rupture of the tendon of long head of biceps (p. 138).

Lesions of the rotator cuff (see Fig. 16.10, p. 136).

RHEUMATOID ARTHRITIS

Rheumatoid arthritis affects connective tissues generally as well as the synovium of joints. Many of the soft tissue lesions so far described can be caused by rheumatoid arthritis. If the symptoms are resistant to treatment this condition should be excluded.

INTERVERTEBRAL DISC DEGENERATION

The normal intervertebral disc contains a nucleus pulposus which consists of a gel-like mucopolysaccharide. This is surrounded by an annulus fibrosus made of fibrous tissue. The disc is separated from the bone of the vertebral body by a layer of hyaline cartilage. Anteriorly it is constrained by the anterior longitudinal ligament and posteriorly by the posterior longitudinal ligament.

The disc alters with age. The water content of the nucleus pulposus is reduced and the protein polysaccharides are altered. The annulus fibrosus changes approximately to fibrocartilage. At the age of sixty, it is difficult to distinguish between the nucleus purposus and the greater part of the annulus. This alteration with age is described as disc degeneration. The majority of people with 'degenerative' discs do not complain of symptoms. Many people who develop back symptoms do not have any significant disc disease. However, many back syndromes are ascribed to degenerative disc disease. It is found that the material of a disc protrusion through a ruptured annulus is similar to that in an old person's disc. It is widely considered that the first process to occur in patients with disc lesions is this degenerative process. When it has occurred the patient is liable to various mechanical malfunctions and symptoms result (Fig. 12.3). Probably the earliest of these is the Schmorl's node, which is considered to result from a rupture of the hyaline cartilage plate between the disc and the vertebral body. It is seen as a small circular radiolucent area on X-ray.

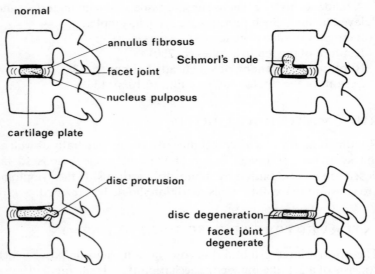

Fig. 12.3   Intervertebral disc lesions.

Cracks can also occur in the annulus fibrosus and this will permit material from the nucleus to escape posteriorly. If sufficient material escapes an adjacent nerve root may be involved and nerve root symptoms of sciatica result.

The disc will lose its turgor as a result of these lesions and no longer act as an efficient buffer. It tends to collapse, which throws strain on the relevant intervertebral facet joints, and also on the posterior ligaments of the spine, causing the symptoms of back ache. A collapsed disc with strained or even subluxed facet joints at one segment indicates that the segment is weakened. Quite minor trauma can cause severe back pain which may be incapacitating. These patients are subject to severe episodes of back pain after heavy work or after lifting awkwardly, or after sudden twisting movements. They suffer from the syndrome of 'instability' in that particular intervertebral segment.

Over the years, overt secondary degenerative changes will occur in the facet joints and osteophytes will be produced. These, in association with narrowing of the disc space and thickening of the posterior ligaments, will cause narrowing of the vertebral canal (vertebral stenosis) and narrowing of the nerve root foramen (which causes symptoms of nerve root compression).

CHAPTER 13

Neurological Lesions and Orthopaedic Surgery

Patients with neurological signs may have disabilities and deformities requiring orthopaedic treatment. These disabilities and deformities include:

Contracture of muscles
A completely denervated muscle atrophies and in due course is replaced by fibrous tisue. This may shorten and produce a contracture.

Joint contractures
Collagen is laid down along lines of stress. If a joint is immobile the stress lines will congeal in a certain direction, collagen will be laid down and a contracture result.

Deformities due to muscle imbalance
In many neurological lesions, the paralysis of a limb is incomplete. The activity of some muscles is no longer counteracted by their antagonists. The limb is liable to be forced into abnormal postures by these unopposed muscles and in due course a deformity will result. On occasions this process can result in subluxation or dislocation of a joint.

Lesions due to loss of touch and pain sensation
Areas of skin will lose protective sensibility and damage can result from unperceived trauma. Denervation of skin also results in loss of the bulk of subcutaneous tissues, loss of sweating and nail atrophy. These are known as trophic disturbances.

Disability due to loss of position sense
Patients with a denervated limb also lose any awareness of its position in space. This is found in patients with spinal cord lesions and to some extent in patients with cerebral palsy. This loss of position sense greatly decreases the function of the paretic limb and makes rehabilitation very difficult. Neuropathic joints are liable to develop in patients with impaired position sense.

Disuse osteoporosis
This occurs in paretic limbs.

Growing children with neurological abnormalities are especially liable to develop deformities:
1. Overall bone growth will be inhibited and the affected limb will be short.
2. The epiphysis will be affected by abnormal forces and deformities result from abnormal growth.
3. The effects of muscle imbalance and contractures are accentuated and deformities tend to progress relentlessly.
4. Scoliosis may result from abnormalities of back muscles.

PERIPHERAL NERVE LESIONS

Peripheral nerve injuries are classified as to their severity (Fig. 13.1).

Neuropraxia
This is a benign disturbance of nerve function lasting a few days. It is a physiological interruption of peripheral nerve function. The lesion is often incomplete with motor paralysis but some residual sensory function.

Axonotmesis
The nerve fibres are damaged sufficiently for the individual axons to degenerate. However the endoneural tubes remain intact so that complete recovery can occur. This type of lesion is common with fractures.

Neurotmesis
This indicates either actual anatomical division of the nerve or severe scarring such that spontaneous regeneration is impossible.

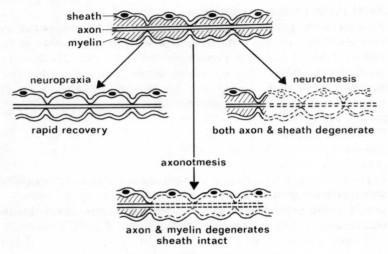

Fig. 13.1   Peripheral nerve injury.

Surgical repair is required. This type of lesion occurs with lacerations, and after severe traction injuries or ischaemia.

After section a nerve fibre undergoes Wallerian degeneration, which involves:

1. Degeneration of the axon.

2. Breaking up of the myelin sheath.

3. Narrowing of the endoneural tubes.

4. In due course, deterioration of the muscle end/plates and atrophy of the muscle fibres. The sensory endings also become atrophied.

The reparative process is as follows:

1. Debris is removed by macrophages.

2. Fibroblasts enter the gap and form fibrous tissue. The Schwann cells of the endoneural tube proliferate and cross the gap to reform the endoneural tubes. If the gap is too large fibrous tissue predominates and it cannot be bridged by the proliferating Schwann cells.

3. Axon fibrils grow down the spaces between the Schwann cells and traverse the lesion to enter the distal endoneural tube. They will eventually reach the end organs.

4. New myelin sheath is developed and nerve function returns. This process takes several months.

Acute peripheral nerve injuries

All patients suffering lacerations or fractures should be suspected of
having nerve lesions., They should be purposefully examined to
exclude them. The movements subserved by the relevant muscles
should be tested, although this may be difficult in patients with
painful injured limbs.

Sensation should be tested. In recently injured patients, gross pin
prick is probably the most useful.

Any laceration which is likely to involve a nerve should be
explored by a formal operation with tourniquet and general
anaesthesia. A laceration on the volar aspect of the wrist is best
treated this way since either or both median and ulnar nerves can be·
damaged from such an injury. Lesions associated with fractures are
usually either neuropraxia or axonotmesis. Such lesions are usually
recoverable and do not require operation, but if not they must be
explored.

Late peripheral nerve injury

These require careful and painstaking examination which should
include:

1. Examination of the original scar, noting any neuroma or
Tinel's sign.

2. The attitude of the limb; wrist drop is seen in radial nerve
injury, a foot drop with a peroneal nerve injury.

3. Motor function, which includes observation of wasting and
trick movements and an assessment and grading of muscle power.

4. Sensibility – assessment of touch, pain and proprioception
and tactile discrimination.

5. Trophic changes – loss of sweating, loss of skin markings,
pulp atrophy, colour changes, loss of hair or atrophic nails.

6. Testing of reflexes.

7. Noting passive range of movement of relevant joints. These
should be as mobile as possible before operation.

Conservative treatment includes:

Splintage to prevent deformities and overstretching of paralysed
muscles.

Passive exercises to paralysed joints.

Electric stimulation to prevent wasting particularly of small
muscles of the hand.

Operative treatment involves:

Exploration of any open lesion when in doubt as to the integrity of a nerve.

Primary repair, indicated when a good surgeon and good facilities are available and the lesion itself is clean and clearcut.

Secondary repair (after 3 to 6 weeks), indicated when the lesion is dirty or the nerve is damaged over a considerable extent.

A nerve graft, which can be performed if there is a considerable gap in the damaged nerve. The graft can be taken from a cutaneous nerve – the sural nerve is frequently used.

The prognosis of a peripheral nerve injury depends on:

1. The severity of the injury. Complete recovery is the rule with a neuropraxia and is possible with an axonotmesis. Even in the most favourable circumstances, a neurotmesis is often followed by an incomplete recovery.

2. The age. The younger the patient the more perfect the recovery.

3. The site. The more distal the lesion the more perfect the recovery.

4. The time before operation. The earlier the repair the more perfect the recovery.

5. The technique of repair and skill of the surgeon. If an operating microscope is used it is possible to match individual bundles of fibres and place sutures meticulously through the supporting tissues.

NERVE ENTRAPMENT PHENOMENA

A peripheral nerve may be trapped either in an osseo-fibrous tunnel or in a fibrous-edged slit in muscle. The symptoms may be caused either by pressure on the nerve or by interference with its blood supply. Trauma may start the symptoms and persistent inflammation potentiate them.

In general, these patients suffer a persistent burning pain which is worst at night. This is often accompanied by 'pins and needles' and numbness. There may be tenderness at the entrapment site.

Carpal tunnel syndrome (p. 116)

Carpal tunnel syndrome is the commonest of these lesions. It occurs frequently but not exclusively in middle-aged ladies. The carpal tunnel is formed by the flexor retinaculum bridging the carpus. The flexor tendons in their sheaths are contained in the tunnel. Pressure on the median nerve as it passes through the tunnel causes the patients to complain of pain, numbness and tingling predominantly in the index, middle and ring fingers of the affected hand. These symptoms are worse at night on waking and may be relieved by altering the position of the affected limb. There is frequently a feeling of clumsiness on using the hand. On examination there are no definite signs; occasionally some thenar wasting is seen.

Ulnar nerve neuritis (p. 117)
The ulnar nerve passes through a fibro-osseous tunnel behind the medial epicondyle at the elbow. It can be trapped here and symptoms of ulnar nerve neuritis arise.

The deep branch of the ulnar nerve may be trapped as it passes round the hook of the hamate in the hand. This is an uncommon lesion.

Thoracic outlet syndrome
In this condition, the brachial plexus and subclavian artery are compressed as the structures leave the neck for the axilla. Various anatomical sites for such compression have been described.

Cervical rib compression
The lower two roots of the brachial plexus and the subclavian artery can be compressed between the scalenus anterior muscle and the cervical rib with its fibrous extension.

Scalenus anterior syndrome
The lower two roots of the brachial plexus and subclavian artery can be compressed between the scalenus anterior and medius muscles and the first rib.

Costo-clavicular syndrome
The brachial plexus and subclavian artery can be compressed between the clavicle and the first rib.

The patients present with symptoms of pain and numbness and paraesthesia down the arm to the hand. In particular the lower two roots (C8 and T1) of the plexus are affected. Severe cases will have wasting of the small muscles of the hand and sensory loss over the little finger and inner side of the arm.

In addition patients may exhibit Raynaud's phenomenon in the hand, and occasionally more severe vascular changes.

The scalenus anterior syndrome can be confirmed by Adson's manoeuvre of hyperextension of the neck, turning the head to the side of the lesion, and forced inspiration. This may reproduce the hand symptoms and reduce the volume of the radial pulse.

These patients present classically after suddenly performing heavier work than they are used to. Nowadays they are frequently seen after road traffic accidents. Treatment should be conservative as a great many of these patients will recover. It is rational to prescribe exercises (shoulder shrugging) to improve the function of the trapezium and other muscles and thus relieve tension on the brachial plexus. If neurological signs are present and the symptoms persistent the root of the neck can be explored by operation and the source of compression relieved.

Other nerves which may be involved in similar lesions are:
Posterior interosseous nerve as it passes through the supinator.
Obturator nerve through the obturator forearm.
Lateral cutaneous nerve of the thigh through a canal in the inguinal ligament.
Peroneal nerve around the fibula neck. Posterior tibial nerve beneath the flexor retinaculum behind the medial malleolus.

BRACHIAL PLEXUS LESIONS

These are usually traction injuries caused by forced lateral flexion of the head on the trunk. Such injuries can occur during birth but are most frequently seen in adults as a result of motorcycle accidents. The traction injury can cause a neuropraxia, axonotmesis or neurotmesis or frequently a combination of these lesions in the different elements of the plexus. High speed motorcycle accidents can result in actual avulsion of the nerve roots from the cervical spinal cord (Fig. 13.2).

Birth trauma

This may be a benign lesion which recovers completely. The commonest residual lesion is an Erb's palsy and the lesion is stated to occur at Erb's point, the junction of C5 and C6 nerve roots. These patients have a residual paresis of deltoid, of elbow flexors, of supinator and of wrist extensors.

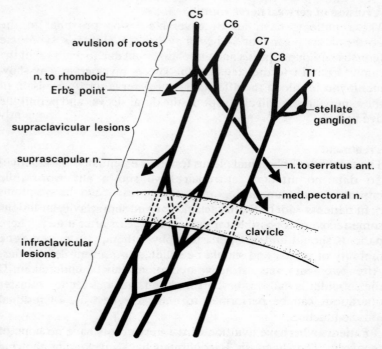

Fig. 13.2 Brachial plexus.

A Klumpke's paralysis is less common and involves C8 and T1 nerve roots causing a paresis of finger flexors and the intrinsic muscles of the hand.

Infraclavicular lesions
These may be associated with a fractured clavicle or dislocated shoulder. The lesion is often incomplete involving cords and nerves and the prognosis for recovery is usually good.

Supraclavicular lesions
These patients frequently have a completely paralysed upper limb, sparing only the rhomboids and serratus anterior. There may be complete sensory loss as well in which case the prognosis for recovery is poor. Recovery however may occur over 1–2 years and it is best not to be dogmatic in assessing these patients.

Avulsion of cervical nerve roots

These patients have an irrecoverable lesion proximal to the posterior root ganglion. They may have a Horner's syndrome (constricted pupil, ptosis and enophthalmos) due to avulsion of the ramus from T1 to the stellate ganglion. A myelogram may show meningoceles along the affected cervical nerve roots. Avulsion of these nerve roots will also rupture the dural sleeves and permit the dye to leak.

Treatment

The treatment of brachial plexus lesions is essentially conservative. To date no attempts at repair have shown any worthwhile improvement of function.

In patients with birth, infraclavicular and supraclavicular lesions some recovery is possible for at least two years after injury. These patients should undergo persistent physiotherapy to preserve the mobility of joints, and should be splinted to prevent deformities. After two years, reconstructive operations may be undertaken. If the shoulder is flail it is best arthrodesed. Various tendon transfer operations can be performed to make the best use of residual muscle function.

Patients who have avulsion of the nerve roots have no hope of recovery. The diagnosis is confirmed by a myelogram showing meningoceles. These patients are probably best treated by providing them with a specially designed lightweight brachial plexus splint. On occasion the limb has been so painful that amputation has been advised.

PARAPLEGIA AND TETRAPLEGIA

The majority of these cases result from trauma. Other conditions such as multiple sclerosis, ascending myelitis, tumours and infections can produce a more gradual progressive lesion.

Fractures of the dorsal spine with significant displacement almost inevitably produce a complete paraplegia, as the vertebral canal is so narrow in this region. These patients have a complete paralysis of their lower limbs. Initially this paralysis is flaccid (a state of 'spinal shock') but over a period of weeks it converts to a spastic paralysis. Reflex activity returns to the intact segments of the spinal cord distal to the lesion (Fig. 13.3). There is complete sensory loss. All

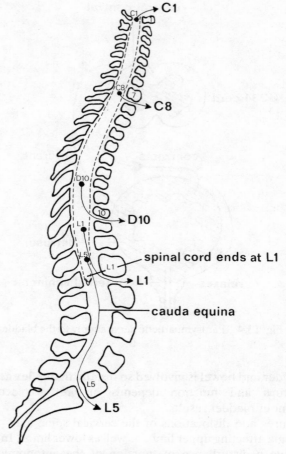

Fig. 13.3 Relationship of the spinal cord to the vertebrae.

modalities are affected, touch, pain, and position sense. In a complete lesion there will be no recovery for these modalities.

There is initially complete loss of bladder and bowel function. After a few weeks, reflex activity returns, resulting in an automatic bladder (Fig. 13.4).

Fractures of the lumbar spine will only cause neurological lesions if they are grossly displaced. These lesions are incomplete and will affect the nerve roots of the cauda equina (the spinal cord ends at the level of the first lumbar vertebra in adults). The nerve supply to

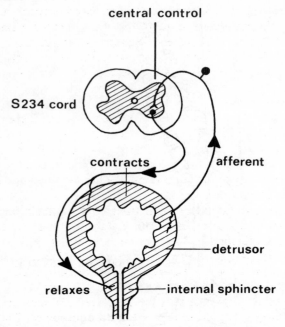

Fig. 13.4   Parasympathetic nerve supply to the bladder.

the bladder and bowel is involved so distally that reflex activity will not return and function depends on intrinsic activity – an autonomous bladder results.

Fractures and dislocations of the cervical spine may produce a tetraplegia affecting upper limbs as well as lower limbs. In addition, they have a disturbance of function of the autonomic nervous system; they may develop paralytic ileus or a profound hypotension.

The severity of the lesion of the upper limbs depends on the level of the injury to the cervical spine. A patient with an injury at C3–4 level may well have no function in the upper limbs and require assisted respiration in order to survive. The commonest lesion is at C5–6 level. At this level the C6 nerve root may or may not be functional and the residual capacity varies accordingly.

A patient who is completely paraplegic on admission will probably show no neurological recovery. Unfortunately, at present, no form of treatment will alter this.

A patient with an incomplete lesion may improve. A careful neurological examination should be made to detect any signs of an incomplete lesion such as toe movement or sparing of sacral sensation. Operative decompression of the spinal cord is only indicated if an incomplete lesion appears to be getting worse.

Initial management
It is essential not to inflict further damage on moving these patients. They should be carried in 'one straight piece' with the spine extended at the fracture. Three persons are required to lift and one more is necessary to supervise. Four people are required to lift a tetraplegic patient – the supervisor holding the head and keeping the neck in extension.

These patients ideally should travel flat on their backs with pressure areas supported by pillows and the fracture maintained in extension. Unfortunately they often have other injuries and in order to maintain a good airway, they can be put in a modified coma position with spine straight and supported with pillows.

Care of the skin must start immediately. These people rapidly develop pressure sores as they are paralysed and have no pain or touch sensation. The position should be changed every 2 hours and pressure points protected.

The fractures are usually managed consevatively. Those of the dorsal and lumbar spine can be reduced by hyperextension over pillows and maintained adequately. Fractures and dislocations of the cervical spine can be reduced by skull traction and the reduction so maintained. Skull traction is via tongs inserted into the outer table of the skull. These patients can be treated on a turning bed. Only patients with gross malalignment require open reduction and internal fixation.

The bladder requires care to prevent over-distension of the paralysed detrusor muscle. Catheterisation must be performed under very strict aseptic conditions to prevent infection. It will be some weeks before a reflex bladder can empty itself.

Definitive management
Definitive management of paraplegic patients requires a centre with proper facilities and staff. These people require special nursing and rehabilitation. The overall prognosis has improved dramatically since the need for better facilities has been appreciated.

Meticulous care of the skin is essential to prevent sores. These patients in the early stages require turning every 2 hours; this demands either a three man team or a special turning bed. Pressure sores once present are very difficult to eradicate. Furthermore they will initiate reflex spasms and cause postural problems and eventually contractures. A patient in a wheelchair must be taught to change his position every hour to prevent pressure sores. Particular care must be taken in fitting footwear and any special appliances.

The bladder must be retrained. After injury the detrusor muscle is completely paralysed; in due course reflex contractions will return but there will be no central control. The patient can learn to initiate the contraction in various ways. Ideally there should be as low a residual urine as possible.

Bladder training involves:

1. Regular catheterisation (or use of an indwelling catheter) until a reflex bladder is established.

2. The avoidance of infection in the urinary tract.

3. Rapid treatment of infection when it occurs.

4. Establishment of a reflex bladder with as low a residual urine as possible.

5. The control of incontinence.

Unfortunately most patients have some residual bladder and bowel problems. These are very severe in those with a persistently paralysed or autonomous bladder (as seen in those with cauda equina lesions).

These patients initially have a complete paralysis of bowel function. They require persistent treatment with enemas and manual evacuation until reflex activity returns. When this happens it is possible for the patient to learn how to stimulate reflex defaecation.

Intensive physiotherapy is necessary to prevent contractures and deformities by daily passive movement of all joints, careful positioning of paralysed limbs, and splinting. It helps the development of upper limb and trunk muscles once the initial fracture has stabilised. This has to be done gradually to avoid problems of postural hypotension. These muscles are developed to permit sitting, to allow transfer from bed to wheelchair and to allow standing in braces to help kidney and bowel function.

Tetraplegic patients may have problems with respiratory function requiring treatment.

Rehabilitation means adaptation
of the patient to his disability,

of the patient's residual capacities to new functions, and

of the patient's environment to accommodate him. His waking hours will be spent predominantly in a wheelchair which can be adapted to his needs. His house and garden must be adapted to accommodate him. If his employer will not accept him, the patient can be trained in skills that will be accepted. Certain recreations are denied him, so he is taught new ones.

POLIOMYELITIS

Poliomyelitis is a virus disease which affects the anterior horn cells of the spinal cord. Fortunately it is now uncommon in Western countries due to the success of immunisation programmes. There are still many patients showing the residue of the disease (Fig. 13.5).

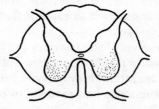

Fig. 13.5 Poliomyelitis affects anterior horn cells.

The anterior horn cells are damaged and a lower motoneurone lesion with no sensory loss results. The patient will have:

Paresis limited to certain muscle groups.

Flaccid muscles which may atrophy and be replaced by fibrous tissue.

Absent or decreased tendon reflexes.

The development of contractures and deformities.

Deformities occur in poliomyelitis because:

1. Contractures will develop around motionless joints.

2. Paralysed muscles will be replaced by fibrous tissue, which will contract.

3. Some muscles are affected more than others. As a result, there will be an imbalance between the protagonist and antagonist muscles of a particular movement; abnormal movement and deformity result. In some cases, joints will be subluxed or even dislocated.

4. The spine may be affected by muscle imbalance and scoliosis result.

5. In children, shortening will occur due to diminished bone growth of paretic limbs.

6. In children, the shape of bones may be altered by loss of normal muscled activity. For example, the gluteus medius and minimus muscles which abduct the hip joint are attached to the greater trochanter. If they are weak the greater trochanter and outer side of the femoral neck will lose its normal stimulus for growth. The greater trochanter will be small and the neck shaft angle increased resulting in coxa valga (see Fig. 3.3).

Treatment

In the acute stage treatment involves splintage for paralysed limbs and passive movements for joints.

In the convalescent stage muscles are rehabilitatd by active exercises. Splintage is required to support flail limbs and prevent contractures.

After about one year very little recovery can be expected and the patient may be left with a residual paralysis. Splintage is required to support flail limbs. Operations may improve function and include:

1. The release of muscles and tendons to correct contractures and deformities.

2. Muscle and tendon transfers to make the best use of undamaged muscles and to prevent them acting as a deforming force.

3. Stabilising operations (usually joint arthrodesis) for unstable segments of the limb. At the same time a deformity can be corrected.

4. Operative correction with rods and spinal fusion for scoliosis, which can be severe.

5. Leg lengthening operations, if discrepancy in leg length is great enough to justify it.

MYELOMENINGOCELE

These patients present with a plaque of damaged spinal cord on the surface of the skin (Fig. 13.6). In some this is enclosed in a cyst. The plaque is usually in the lumbar or thoracolumbar regions. Unless this lesion is closed, they are liable to die from infection. It has

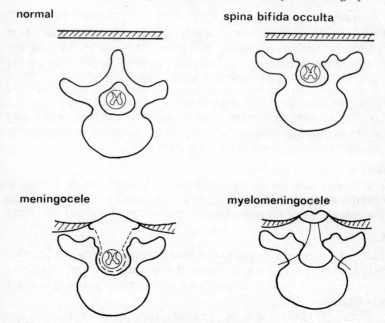

Fig. 13.6 Spina bifida, meningocele and myelomeningocele.

become policy to close these lesions and treat the patients with antibiotics.

These patients have several general problems:

1. A complete or incomplete paralysis of the lower limbs.

2. Often multiple deformities of the lower limbs.

3. No active control of bladder function and a tendency to develop renal failure.

4. Often hydrocephalus requiring surgical relief.

5. Often other associated brain abnormalities.

They are frequently ill and frequently mentally retarded. Their general health is poor. They present very difficult orthopaedic problems.

Paralysis

This paralysis can be complete or incomplete. Usually there is a flaccid paralysis but a spastic paralysis can exist in segments distal to the lesion.

Deformities
Deformities occur because of paralysis and muscle imbalance. They tend to become worse as the child grows. Because both flaccid and spastic paresis can exist in the same patient, deformities due to muscle imbalance can occur in a totally paralysed patient.

Problems associated with sensory loss
Trophic lesions can occur, and great care must be taken with footwear and splintage. Loss of proprioception decreases the function expected from the level of paralysis.

Bones
The bones are small, osteoporotic and deformed and tend to fracture easily. The legs are short and, in some patients, leg length discrepancy requires correction.

Vertebrae
The vertebrae are congenitally abnormal and scoliosis or other deformities may occur. These frequently require operative correction as a straight stable back is necessary in order to use a wheelchair.

These patients are assessed neurologically as soon as possible and the assessment repeated. A prognosis of eventual capabilities depends on the neurological level of the lesion. The prognosis also depends on the general health and mental capabilities of the child. A patient who is totally paralysed – a T12 lesion with no active movement in the lower limbs – will use a wheelchair as an adult. As a child, he may 'ambulate' with long braces and pelvic harness swinging through with crutches. Such a gait is good exercise but not economical or practical.

A patient with an L4 lesion will have good quadriceps function. In due course he may walk with below-knee bracing and support his hips with sticks or crutches. Such ambulation is functional, practical and may be economical. Patients with lower lesions will have an even better prognosis.

Treatment
Conservative treatment
1. The prevention of deformities by physiotherapy and splintage.
2. Special training to stand and to walk to the best of their ability, involving graduated splintage.
3. Careful supervision of splintage. As the child grows he will

outgrow his splint. There is loss of pain sensation so fitting must be meticulous to prevent trophic ulcers. Loss of touch is important as it is necessary for the patient to feel the splint to be aware of it. Elaborate splints are required for patients with loss of touch sensation. There is loss of proprioception, and splintage will have to extend proximal to any denervated joint in order to compensate for this.

Operative treatment
This follows much the same lines as that for poliomyelitis; however the results are not so dramatic.

Operations for foot deformities are of particular importance. Practically every deformity can occur in patients with myelomeningocele. In young patients, a soft tissue correction can be performed. In older patients bony operations are necessary.

The hip is particularly at risk with an L4 lesion. These patients will have no active hip abductors or extensors but will have active flexors and adductors. These muscles will tend to dislocate the hip. This can be prevented by transferring the ilio-psoas complex through the blade of the ilium to the greater trochanter so that it acts as an abductor and will stabilise the hip joint.

Back deformities present a difficult problem in patients with spina bifida and operation is frequently required for these.

Cord tethering
Other less severe spine lesions can cause less severe neurological problems. Spina bifida is common. There are usually no signs or symptoms but X-ray will reveal a bifid lumbar spine. This may be associated with overlying skin discolouration or a hairy patch. This may be complicated by an intravertebral lipoma or a diastematomyelia (a bone deformity which may split the spinal cord). Either of these lesions may cause tethering of the spinal cord. The vertebral canal grows faster than the spinal cord in children so the cord tends to 'rise', but if it is tethered a traction lesion will develop in the roots of the cauda equina. Deformities or weakness of the lower limbs will result. Pes cavus (a high arched foot) is the most frequent. Associated with this will be bladder disturbances such as enuresis.

CEREBRAL PALSY

Cerebral palsy is an inclusive term to describe non-progressive disorders of the brain in young children which cause impairment of motor function. In addition, there is impairment of position sense and frequently diminished mental capacity and emotional disturbances.

It is a relatively common condition. Often there is no identifiable cause. The known causes can be listed:

Prenatal
   Heredity
   Prematurity
   Some lesions of pregnancy – toxaemia or antepartum haemorrhage
   Kernicterus or hydrocephalus
Natal (occurring at birth)
   Abnormal labour or fetal anoxia
Postnatal
   Trauma
   Meningitis or other severe infections of infancy.

These children have varying physical signs as they develop and the clinical picture alters. The diagnosis is difficult in the early stages but various factors indicate the diagnosis:

Excessive sleepiness
Difficulty with feeding (particularly sucking)
Abnormal posture
Delayed milestones, especially sitting and walking

Spasticity
The majority of cerebral palsy children exhibit spasticity. This means that the limb muscles have increased tone. The lesion is said to occur in the motor cortex or pyramidal tracts.

Some muscle groups are more spastic than others and some are weaker than others. Imbalance of muscle function results and deformities occur. These patients may be helped by operations.

Athetosis
These patients have persistent writhing movements and also may have some degree of spasticity. The lesion is in the basal ganglia. Some deformities may be relieved by operation but athetoids are rarely suitable on account of emotional instability.

Ataxia
Some patients exhibit gross ataxia and these are considered to have lesions of the cerebellum. Operations are rarely indicated.

Hemiplegia

These patients have a unilateral spastic paresis. The upper limb is often more severely affected and held in a classical position to the side with the elbow and wrist flexed and the forearm pronated.

Diplegia

These patients have a spastic paresis affecting the lower limbs more severely than the upper limbs.

Bilateral hemiplegia

These patients have a spastic paresis involving all four limbs; the upper limbs are affected most severely. They often have an associated severe mental defect.

Treatment

The management of these patients is difficult and requires the help of various specialists. Careful assessment is required of general defects. Intelligence tests are necessary. The emotional state is important. The social background should be thoroughly investigated. Special tests are required to detect hearing and visual defects.

Treatment is best accomplished in a special centre where regular physiotherapy, training for daily living and particular educational facilities are available.

Physiotherapy is directed to improving balance and developing co-ordination.

Muscle relaxation can be supervised and weak muscles developed. Prevention of deformities by manipulation and splintage is important. The children require splintage when young to support their paretic limbs and encourage mobility. The deformities can sometimes be prevented by splintage and those already corrected can be maintained.

These patients must be carefully assessed before operation as the results can be variable. In particular they are liable to exacerbate emotional disturbances or social maladjustments. Operations are advised:

1. To relieve deformities by release of contractures of muscles and joints.

2. To prevent deformities by decreasing the activity of overactive muscles. This can be done by operative release or selective denervation (neurectomy).

3. To stabilise a joint by arthrodesis.
4. To correct scoliosis.

Equinus is a deformity of the foot and ankle, which will not dorsiflex to a right angle and permit the heel to reach the ground. This requires surgical correction to lengthen the tendo achilles. Patients frequently have *over-active* hip *adductor muscles* and will exhibit scissoring. If this persists, a valgus deformity of the neck of the femur or even a 'paralytic' dislocation of the hip can result. If the child has tight adductors (with an abduction in extension of less than 20°) they should be released and possibly an anterior obturator neurectomy performed.

Operations on the upper limbs may improve the appearance but rarely affect function. These patients frequently have little postural control over their upper limbs.

Upper motoneuron lesions in adults

Motoneuron lesions occur frequently as a result of trauma, cerebrovascular accidents, subarachnoid haemorrhage, multiple sclerosis and numerous other lesions. These people can be extensively rehabilitated by patient and dedicated therapists. In some ways this rehabilitation is easier than that of cerebral palsy children as these patients already know what they have to achieve.

Upper limb function is best improved by splintage and intensive occupational and physiotherapy. Operations are rarely of value.

In the lower limb, intensive conservative treatment is essential. Splintage may be required for an unstable foot or ankle. A drop foot with weak peronei is fairly frequently found in a stroke patient and can be well-accommodated in a polypropylene splint.

Operations should be performed if indicated. A patient with an equinus deformity will have difficulty in fitting any orthotic appliance. A tendo achilles lengthening may help considerably. A young patient with an unstable equino-varus foot will certainly benefit from stabilisation by a triple arthrodesis to such an extent as to be able to discard lower limb splintage. Adduction contracture of the hips is seen in paraparetic patients such as those with multiple sclerosis. This contracture can be released in combination with an obturator neurectomy. Such an operation will make the patient more comfortable and his nursing care much easier.

CHAPTER 14

Treatment of Orthopaedic Patients

The orthopaedic patient attends with symptoms of pain, disability or deformity. He wishes relief from these symptoms and requires reassurance that they are not indicative of some serious disease. He also requires reassurance that the symptoms will not become more severe.

Treatment therefore involves not only relieving his symptoms, but also reassuring him. Some patients' fears regarding prognosis are excessive and irrational. These people are described as having a 'large functional element' or as being psychosomatic. However, it must be realised that every patient has a functional element to some degree; it is only the proportion of this functional element that varies. It is important for a doctor not to be surprised or irritated about this. One must accept that it is there and treat it as such.

In order to relieve symptoms, it is necessary to make an accurate diagnosis. Sometimes this is easy; sometimes it is impossible. However it is often possible to exclude any serious disease and reassure the patient accordingly.

The diagnosis involves taking a history, clinical examination, X-rays, blood tests, and special investigations. Routine diagnostic measures involve the relevant plain X-rays and blood tests. Special investigations may be very expensive, or the facilities required may not be available. Some special investigations are invasive and are liable to cause symptoms on their own account. It requires judgement and experience to determine if such investigations are necessary.

For a few orthopaedic conditions, there are specific lines of treatment which are generally accepted as being necessary, e.g. a patient with acute osteomyelitis requires specific treatment in order to relieve his symptoms and cure the condition. However, the majority of orthopaedic conditions can be managed in varying ways depending on the patient, the experience of his doctor, and the degree and the severity of the condition.

Even a patient with a specific condition such as osteosarcoma may be treated in varying ways. The prognosis of this condition is so poor that it is reasonable to discuss possible treatment with the patient. In conditions such as osteoarthritis of the hip, treatment depends on the patient's age, his necessary activities and his psychological make-up.

The treatment of low back pain involves so many variables that even though it is such a common condition, the management is completely bewildering and in some cases is quite irrational.

The majority of orthopaedic patients suffer from chronic conditions such as degenerative disease or rheumatoid arthritis. These patients suffer from episodic symptoms, having relapses and remissions of the pain. This is particularly so with rheumatoid arthritis. Osteoarthritic patients with degenerative changes in their joints suffer exacerbations of symptoms following excessive use or even minor trauma. Treatment of the patient's symptoms resulting from these exacerbations will make him much more comfortable. Such treatment will not cure the underlying condition. A patient with osteoarthritis of the knee can be made much more comfortable by a short period of treatment with rest, bandaging and anti-inflammatory and analgesic drugs.

The treatment of orthopaedic conditions may involve:
'No treatment'
Drugs
Physiotherapy and occupational therapy
Traction
Rest
Orthoses
Operations

'No treatment'

There are many patients who attend with symptoms of pain in the back or limbs for which no cause can be found on clinical examination or by simple investigations. These patients will benefit from being reassured that no identifiable lesion is discovered and that there is no evidence of any serious cause of their condition such as infection or tumours or 'arthritis'.

When reassuring these patients, it is best to emphasise that they have not got 'arthritis' or a 'slipped disc'. These lesions are recognised by the general public as being incurable and as proceeding inevitably to crippling and deformity.

Drugs

Drug treatment for orthopaedic conditions should, if possible, be directed either towards relief of exacerbations of a chronic disease such as arthritis, or to specific management of a specific condition.

Drugs such as sulphinpyrazone or colchicine are used for gout. Gold is of value in rheumatoid arthritis. Antibiotics are used to combat specific infections. Drugs are also used non-specifically to treat the exacerbations of chronic degenerative conditions and rheumatoid arthritis. They will not usually affect the progress of the condition. Aspirin is both an analgesic and an anti-inflammatory drug and is exceedingly useful. However most patients will have tried aspirins before consulting their doctor. If they are prescribed simple aspirin they will feel cheated.

Physiotherapy and occupational therapy

Physiotherapists and occupational therapists have an invaluable part to play in the treatment of patients with orthopaedic diseases. They should be given a goal for each patient; the methods should be left to them to decide.

Traction

Traction is used to overcome painful muscle spasm and thus relieve pain. It is also used as a form of splintage to prevent excessive motion. In treatment of fractures, traction can be used to reduce the displaced fragments. The types of traction to be considered are:

Skin traction
Skeletal traction
Traction using a Thomas splint
Other special forms of traction
Skull traction

Skin traction involves the use of strapping extensions on the lower limbs. The extensions are of Elastoplast and the adhesiveness is assisted by the use of tinct.benz.co. The simplest sort of skin traction is that used for patients with back pain and sciatica. The patient lies flat in bed with the end of the bed raised and a weight applied to the affected limb by the use of skin traction. This traction does not have any effect on the disc space but it does relieve the patient's muscle spasm and also ensure that he stays in bed and thus obtains complete bed rest. Skin traction is also used frequently in treating children with various conditions. A gallows traction suspends the legs vertically via skin extensions, with the weight attached to a pulley. This sort of traction is used for treating fractured femurs in very small children and initially in the treatment of congenital dislocation of the hip (Fig. 14.1).

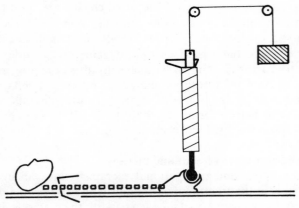

Fig. 14.1　Gallows traction.

Skeletal traction involves the use of a pin placed through the bone. In adults the upper end of the tibia is usually used; the pin is inserted in close relation to the tibial tubercle. This has the advantage of permitting greater weight to be applied to the limb and also it is more permanent as skin extensions tend to peel off after a few weeks. It must be remembered that in growing children the pin should never be placed near the tibial tubercle as this is an actively growing epiphyseal plate. Other sites for skeletal traction are the lower end of the femur, the lower end of the tibia and the calcaneus.

The Thomas splint was devised for treating fractures of the femur. It consists of a leather ring at its upper end which is designed to fit snugly around the groin and impinge on the ischial tuberosity. Attached to this are metal extensions joined at the lower end which fit on either side of the lower leg and below the foot. Traction can be applied either via skin extensions or via a skeletal pin and the cords are tied to the ends of the Thomas splint. This forms a closed system

force transmitted to buttock

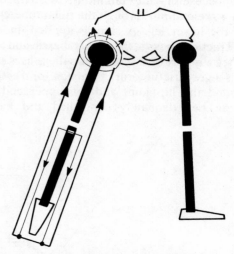

Fig. 14.2   Fixed skeletal traction in Thomas splint.

(Fig. 14.2) and traction from the cords is transmitted back up the lower limb to the groin and the tuberosity via the bars of the Thomas splint. The patient with a limb immobilised in this way can be transported quite comfortably and simply. The Thomas splint is used in various ways and in hospital a variety of systems have been devised to apply traction most efficiently using the Thomas splint as the basis of the apparatus (Fig. 14.3).

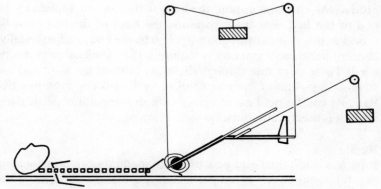

Fig. 14.3   Sliding traction with Thomas splint.

Other forms of traction are used particularly in the lower limbs. One of the most useful is the Hamilton-Russell traction. This can be applied via a skeletal pin through the tibial tubercle. A support is applied to the lower leg. A sling is applied under the thigh to support it. Traction goes via the tibial tubercle and also towards the end of the leg support by a system of pulleys as is shown in Figure 14.4. This is a very useful form of traction for treating people with lesions around the hip joint and the upper end of the femur. Rotation can be adequately controlled and the apparatus is comfortable.

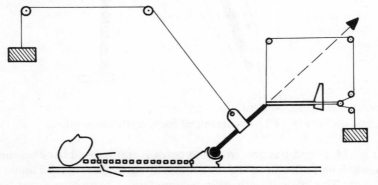

Fig. 14.4   Adapted Hamilton-Russell traction.

Lesions of the neck such as a fracture of the cervical spine or patients with severe pain from cervical spondylosis can be treated by *head traction*. This can be applied by means of a halter which fits around the chin and around the head with a weight applied to the end of the bed. For these patients, the head of the bed must be raised so that counter traction is applied by the body sliding distally. If more permanent traction is required, then skull calipers can be used. These perforate through the outer table of the skull and can remain in position for a matter of several weeks or even months. Patients can be held quite rigidly with this apparatus particularly when it is used in combination with a turning bed.

Rest

Rest is a traditional and very effective method of treating acutely painful conditions. It is particularly useful in treating acute inflammatory lesions, and lesions which follow minor or repetitive trauma. Bed rest is the only really effective method of treating back pain. The hip joint can be rested by bed rest and traction to the affected limb. More distal lesions of the lower limb can be rested by immobilisation in plaster. Rest of the upper limb involves the use of a sling. The elbow or the wrist joint can be immobilised in plaster.

However, bed rest can have disadvantages:

Osteoporosis

Joint stiffness

Muscle atrophy

Thrombotic complications such as deep vein thrombosis or pulmonary embolus

Hypostatic infections of chest or urinary tract

Bed sores

Psychiatric disturbances, particularly of the elderly.

ORTHOTICS

An orthosis may be a splint, a dynamic splint, or a caliper. Orthoses are devised by orthotists and are prescribed by doctors.

Ideally an orthosis is made for a patient's specific disability. They are not designed to treat any particular disease such as cerebral palsy or poliomyelitis.

Orthoses are used:

1. To prevent movement (immobilisation). This involves simple splints (including plaster of paris splints) such as are used for the treatment of trauma, fractures and infections.

2. To limit motion to normal movements. Such orthoses are used to control flail limbs and unstable joints.

3. To prevent deformities. Many deformities are caused by neuromuscular imbalance. Patients with a neurological lesion of sudden onset can benefit from orthotic treatment to prevent deformities occurring from such imbalance. One of the most disabling of such deformities is the hyperflexion of the wrist which occurs after cerebrovascular accidents, which can sometimes be prevented by using a simple cock-up plastic splint. Orthoses are also used to prevent recurrence of deformities after surgical correction.

4. To attempt to correct deformities. In general, a fixed deformity in an adult cannot be corrected by an orthosis. In a child (if there is still potential for bone growth) it is possible to apply forces to obtain a correction. Tibial torsion (presenting with an intoe gait) can be corrected by a Dennis Browne splint. The Dennis

Browne splint is also used to treat club feet, correcting milder forms and improving the appearance of more severe forms.

5. For specific purposes. There are numerous splints for holding hips reduced in babies in the condition of congenital dislocation. Perthes' disease can be treated by a variety of methods; the basis of many of them is to hold the hips in abduction and internal rotation.

6. To compensate for weakness. This occurs predominantly in neuro-muscular conditions. Patients with weakness of dorsiflexors of the foot will tend to develop a plantar flexion deformity. Various spring-loaded appliances have been devised so that the energy of plantar flexion can be stored and used to produce dorsiflexion of the foot while walking. These range from a simple polypropylene drop-foot appliance to more complicated spring-loaded devices.

Disadvantages
Various factors mitigate against the efficient use of orthoses.

Associated sensory loss
Patients with loss of touch sensation will need a splint that will fit far more proximally than would be required to compensate only for motor loss, because they cannot feel the splint. Patients with loss of proprioception are also very much handicapped. This is probably even more so in the upper limb than the lower limb. It is found that many patients with lesions of the cerebral cortex following strokes or patients with cerebral palsy have such a severe loss of proprioception that there is no way of obtaining efficient function of the upper limb. Fitting an orthosis or operative correction may improve the appearance of the upper limb cosmetically; however there will be no functional improvement as there is no sense of position in space.

Contractures
Fixed contractures of a limb are liable to occur after disuse. In the lower limbs this will cause alteration of the centre of gravity and make it very difficult to fit an orthosis efficiently. A paraplegic patient with a fixed flexion contracture of his hips will have his centre of gravity thrown forward and there is no way that any orthosis can be fitted which will allow him to stand up without support from his upper limbs. Equinus deformity in the foot will prevent efficient fitting of an orthosis on the upper limb until corrected by surgery.

Gross deformities
Minor degrees of deformity can nowadays be accommodated in modern orthoses. Modern techniques are so advanced that a certain degree of deformity can be accommodated and the orthosis still be efficient. However severe degrees of deformity cannot be accommodated and such patients may well need operative correction before fitting.

Patient acceptance
It is sometimes very difficult to convince a patient that an orthosis will help him. To some extent this lack of acceptance is the fault of the orthotist, if the patient is fitted with a heavy, cumbersome and ugly appliance. However, usually it is the fault of the prescribing doctor who has failed to detect and treat the psychological component of the patient's symptoms. It is necessary to demonstrate to the patient the value of the orthosis before he will accept it.

Painful conditions
Acutely painful conditions can be treated with an orthosis as a temporary measure while the lesion resolves. Chronically painful lesions cannot be adequately treated by an orthosis and require some other form of treatment to relieve the pain. This is particularly the case with pain in a weight-bearing joint which will only be partially relieved by an orthosis. Other more radical treatment is usually necessary.

ORTHOPAEDIC OPERATIONS

This section is almost a glossary of orthopaedic operations.

A *tenotomy* is simple division of a tendon. This may be closed, but is performed preferably by an open operation. It may relieve a contracture of tendon or muscle or it may diminish its power of contraction (frequently it is performed for both reasons). A tenotomy is frequently performed in patients with neuromuscular imbalance from diseases such as cerebral palsy.

A *tendon* can be *lengthened*. This is also performed to relieve a contracture and diminish muscle power. It is usually performed by a Z lengthening technique as for lengthening the tendo achilles.

A *tendon transfer* permits another muscle to perform the function of the one to which it is transferred. A classical example of a tendon transfer is the use of the extensor indicis to replace the extensor pollicis longus of the thumb.

A *tenodesis* occurs when a tendon is transferred to a new situation across a joint. The tendon acts as a tether only; there is no active muscle function.

Tendon repair can be performed by a variety of techniques. Recently very satisfying technical results have been obtained.

A *tendon graft* is necessary in certain situations. The palmaris longus tendon is used as a graft to replace damaged flexor tendons in the 'no man's land' region of the fingers and palm of the hand.

Lacerated *nerves* are *repaired*. A *primary repair* is performed as soon as possible after injury. It is only feasible if the conditions are ideal and a trained surgeon is available. The operating microscope makes this technically a much more satisfactory procedure. A *secondary nerve repair* is usually performed about six weeks after injury. In these patients the skin wound only is closed primarily, and all infection is resolved. Later a secondary repair is performed; quite adequate results are obtained.

A *nerve graft* can be performed if any large portion of nerve is missing. A cutaneous nerve (e.g. sural nerve) is sacrificed and grafted into the defect.

A *neurolysis* means freeing a nerve from fibrous tissue.

Decompression of a nerve is usually performed to relieve pressure as it runs through a fibro-osseous tunnel. A classical example of this is the operation to relieve pressure on the median nerve in the carpal tunnel.

A *laminectomy* involves removal of the lamina of vertebra to expose spinal cord nerve roots or intervertebral discs (see Fig. 18.12, p. 169). A *fenestration laminectomy* is performed through a small window made by removing ligamentum flavum and a minimal amount of adjacent lamina. This operation can be used for removing a lateral disc protrusion. It has the advantage of destroying the least amount of the protective structures about the spine. A *decompression laminectomy* involves removing the spine and lamina and ligamentum flavum so that the whole dura and associated nerve roots are free. The decompression can be extended to include the nerve root canal. A decompression laminectomy is performed frequently to relieve the vertebral stenosis syndrome. It is also used to treat large disc protrusions and intraspinal tumours and infections.

An *arthrotomy* means an operation to open the joint. It is non-specific term for a non-specific operation.

An *arthroscopy* is a method of endoscopic examination of a joint. It is now used almost routinely in the assessment of the knee joint. A good view is obtained of the supra patella pouch and the articular surfaces of the patella and femoral condyles. The lateral meniscus can usually be seen completely as can the anterior cruciate ligament. The medial meniscus can be seen except for its middle portion. It is a very useful aid to the diagnosis of internal derangements of the knee.

An *arthroplasty* is an operation to reconstruct a joint.

An *excision arthroplasty* involves removing a portion of the joint surfaces and creating a false joint. Keller's operation for bunions is a classical example. In this operation an exostosis is removed from the first metatarsal head and in addition the proximal third or half of the proximal phalanx of the great toe is also removed (see Fig. 21.10, p. 244). The term arthroplasty can also be used when the joint is reconstructed using a prosthetic replacement.

A *capsulorrhaphy* implies tightening or reefing of the joint capsule to make it stable, e.g. the Putti-Platt operation for recurrent dislocation of the shoulder (see Fig. 16.8, p. 134).

A joint *ligament reconstruction* operation may be indicated for an unstable joint. Repair of the medial ligament of the knee can be supplemented by using the tendon of semitendinosus.

An *arthrodesis* is an operation which involves obliteration of a joint so that the bones participating in it are fused together by bone. The indications for arthrodesis are:

1. To eradicate a painful joint.
2. To correct a deformity and hold it corrected.
3. To stabilise an unstable joint.

Having eradicated joint surfaces it is necessary to hold the joint in position whilst the process of arthrodesis takes place. Some years ago compression arthrodesis was devised. It was shown that by compressing two cancellous bone surfaces together more rapid union of arthrodesis occurred. An example of this method is knee arthrodesis using compression clamps (see Fig. 20.11c, p. 227).

A prosthetic replacement involves completely replacing a joint by prosthesis (see Fig. 20.11b, p. 227). The simplest of these involves replacing the joint with a spacer such as the Silastic prosthesis that is used to replace the metacarpophalangeal joint in the finger of a patient with rheumatoid arthritis. In the more complicated weight-bearing joints, it is necessary that the components concerned should have several characteristics:

1. The prosthesis must be firmly fixed to the underlying bone. A loose prosthesis is inevitably painful. The most efficient method of fixing a prosthesis to bone is to use acrylic cement which packs firmly into the microscopic interstices of cancellous bone.

2. The prosthesis must not cause a chemical reaction, or produce an immune response. Its fragments, which occur as a result of wear, must produce only a minimal foreign body reaction.

3. The prosthesis must be strong enough to withstand the stresses imposed upon it without becoming deformed. There must be a minimum of wear from its component parts and it must resist fatigue as far as possible. The components which meet these criteria best at the present time are high density polyethylene plastic with stainless steel.

4. The design of the prosthesis must be adequate for its function. It must be stable and not dislocate. Some prostheses are inherently stable, some depend on the patient's own ligaments and capsule for stability.

5. The two components must have a low co-efficient of friction, so that the stresses across the fixation site of the prosthesis are at a minimum. The prosthesis must not be excessively bulky, and must fit anatomically into its implanted site.

An *osteotomy* is a surgical division of bone performed:

1. To correct a bone deformity (as occurs after a malunited fracture).

2. To realign a joint to alter its weight-bearing characteristics, as with a tibial osteotomy for osteo-arthritis of the knee (see Fig. 20.11a, p. 227).

Operations are frequently performed for *osteomyelitis*. In acute osteomyelitis the bone may be *decompressed* by drilling or by performing a fenestration (making a small window in the bone). A *sequestrectomy* is performed in chronic discharging osteomyelitis in the hope of removing the sequestrum and thus the infected focus to permit the lesion to heal.

Bone grafts
The functions of bone grafts are:
1. To promote union of fractures.
2. To assist arthrodesis of joints.

3. To fill in cavities and bridge defects in bone.
4. To act as bone blocks and limit motion of joints.

Bone grafts can be obtained from a variety of sources:
1. *Autogenous* grafts are taken from the patient himself. There are no problems with immune reactions nor with sterilisation. Some cells from cancellous autogenous grafts can survive in the recipient site.
2. *Homogenous* grafts are taken from the same species. Usually freeze-dried cadaveric bone is used. No cells will survive in the recipient site. These grafts have a limited osteogenic inductive capacity and are slowly substituted by new bone. They may have a useful structural function. Homogenous grafts are freeze-dried and specially sterilised.
3. *Heterogeneous* grafts are taken from other species. Deproteinised ox bone is popularly used. These grafts have a structural function and will act as a scaffold, until slowly substituted by new bone.

The osteocytes in the graft will die (except for some of those in cancellous autogenous grafts) and the dead graft will act as a scaffold for new bone which will form from the viable bone ends and the graft bed and attach itself to the graft.

In due course the graft will be resorbed and be replaced by new bone.

Consolidation and remodelling occur later.

Bone grafts have the capacity to cause the primitive mesenchymal cells of the recipient site to form new bone – a process known as osteogenic induction. Autogenous cancellous grafts show the greatest capacity for osteogenic induction. Heterogenous grafts have practically none; however they will act as a scaffold and have a useful structural function.

Amputations
Amputations of limbs are sometimes necessary. The main indications for amputations are:
Vascular disease
Trauma
Persistent infection
Tumours
The first two are the most common. In general a satisfactory amputation must give maximum residual function with sound

healing, and allow adequate fitting of a prosthesis. Of course in amputation for a tumour, the prime consideration is eradication of the tumour.

Patients with diabetes have problems not only with vascular disease, but also with super-imposed infection. In these patients, by resolving the infection, it is possible to perform a much more conservative amputation than would initially appear to be the case.

In the lower limb, the main consideration after amputation is that the limb should be a stable pillar. If the knee joint can be retained, the patient is much more mobile, and an elderly patient will accept the prosthesis much better. If at all possible, one should conserve the knee joint, and in patients with vascular disease, it is reasonable to perform an arterial graft so that this is possible.

In the upper limb, prosthetic fitting is generally unsatisfactory except for extension prostheses for special purposes. The hand depends to a very large extent on sensory feedback, both of touch and proprioception, for adequate function. In general, therefore, an amputation of the upper limb is made as distal as possible to retain as much normal tissue as is reasonable. The exception to this is amputation of the fingers. A single stiff anaesthetic finger is best amputated through the base of the proximal phalanx. As much of the thumb is conserved as is possible.

CHAPTER 15

Wrist and Hands

HISTORY TAKING

The symptoms complained of include:

1. *Pain*, which may be localised or diffuse. Pain in the hand may be referred from the neck or elsewhere in the upper limb.

2. *Weakness, numbness* and *tingling* in the wrist, hand and fingers. These may arise locally from a region such as a carpal tunnel syndrome or from a more proximal lesion, particularly in the neck.

3. *Loss of movement and stiffness.* Patients with rheumatoid arthritis in particular complain of stiffness in the fingers on waking.

4. *Swellings.* The most common cause is a ganglion.

5. *Deformities* such as contractures or the various deformities seen in rheumatoid athritis.

The history of the injury is important. The patient's occupation and social status must be determined, and his general health must be assessed. In particular, enquiries should be made about other joint lesions.

EXAMINATION OF THE WRIST JOINT

This is best done with the patient sitting and both upper limbs fully exposed. Both wrists should be examined simultaneously.

Inspection

Bony contours, in particular the radial and ulnar styloid processes.

Soft tissue contours: any swellings about the wrist joint.

Wasting of the forearm or of the hand.

Deformities of the wrist; one of the commonest is prominence of

107

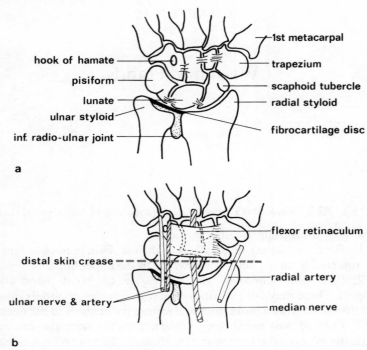

Fig. 15.1 (a) Bony landmarks of right wrist, palmar aspect, (b) structures around right wrist, palmar aspect.

the ulnar styloid due to subluxation of the inferior radio-ulnar joint.
Scars.

Palpation
The bony and soft tissue contours are palpated. Areas of local tenderness should be elicited, in particular over the scaphoid fossa, over the inferior radio-ulnar joint and the tip of the ulnar styloid, over the radial styloid in the region of the abductor pollicis longus and extensor pollicis brevis tendons. Local temperature, radial pulse, skin colour and capillary return should be noted.

Movement
Active and passive movements are measured and compared with the other wrist. The range of dorsiflexion and palmar flexion is

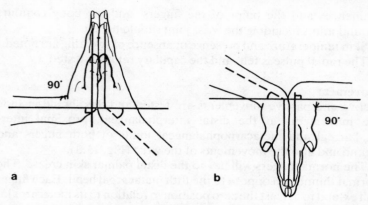

Fig. 15.2 Movements of wrist, (a) limitation of dorsiflexion, (b) limitation of palmar flexion.

about 90° (Fig. 15.2). Rotation movements should be determined with elbows held firmly to the sides. The range is about 80° of pronation and supination. Ulnar and radial deviation should be noted, the range of each being about 25°.

EXAMINATION OF THE HAND

Both hands are compared. Exposure should include both upper limbs.

Inspection

Bony contours of the phalanges and metacarpal bones and the bones of the carpus are noted. Soft tissue contours around joints are examined including any localised swelling or contractures. Any deformities of the fingers of the hand or of the wrist are noted. Any wasting of the thenar or hypothenar or the interossei muscles should be assessed. The first dorsal interosseous is most easily assessed for muscle wasting. Any abnormalities of nails, of pulps of the fingers, alteration in colour or sweating of the skin are noted.

Palpation

The hand should be palpated for local tenderness, particularly around joints.

The soft tissue contours, particularly the thenar and hypothenar eminences and the pulps of the fingers, and the bony contours around joints including the wrist joint should be felt.

Skin temperature and presence or absence of sweating are noted.

The radial pulse is felt, and the capillary return is tested.

Movement

Active and passive movements are tested and this should include the movements at the distal interphalangeal, proximal interphalangeal and metacarpophalangeal joints of both fingers and thumb and also the movements of the wrist (Fig. 15.3).

The normal fingers will flex to the distal palmar skin crease. The normal thumb will oppose to the fifth metacarpal head. Each finger will extend to at least the zero position in relation to its metacarpal.

FLEXION OF FINGERS INTO PALM   EXTENSION OF FINGERS

-of thumb in plane of palm   -of thumb in plane of palm

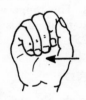

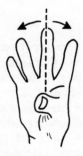

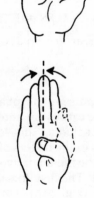

ABDUCTION:
-of fingers from middle fingers
-of thumb at right-angles to palm

ADDUCTION:
-of fingers to middle finger
-of thumb from right-angles to palm

Fig. 15.3   Movements of fingers.

Common deformities of the fingers

Ulnar deviation of one or more fingers at the metacarpophalangeal joint occurs in rheumatoid arthritis.

A *mallet finger* is a flexion deformity of the distal interphalangeal joint of the finger due to damage of the extensor tendon to the distal phalanx (Fig. 15.4). It can usually be passively corrected.

A *boutonnière deformity* is seen at the proximal interphalangeal joint due to loss of the central slip of the extensor tendon. The proximal interphalangeal joint is held flexed and the distal interphalangeal joint extended (Fig. 15.5).

A *swan neck deformity* (Fig. 15.6) is seen in patients with rheumatoid arthritis. This is a hyperextension deformity at the proximal interphalangeal joint accompanied by a flexion deformity at the distal interphalangeal joint. The mechanism is rather complicated.

The *thumb* may be *adducted* into the palm. This is seen in patients with cerebral palsy or after strokes and is a disabling deformity as

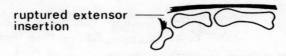

ruptured extensor insertion

Fig. 15.4   Mallet finger deformity.

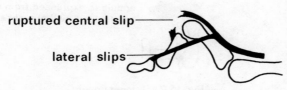

ruptured central slip

lateral slips

Fig. 15.5   Boutonnière deformity.

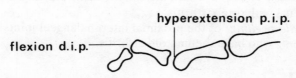

hyperextension p.i.p.

flexion d.i.p.

Fig. 15.6   Swan neck deformity; p.i.p., proximal interphalangeal joint; d.i.p., distal interphalangeal joint.

the thumb is useless and impairs the function of the rest of the hand.

A *claw hand* is seen in ulnar nerve palsy. This involves a hyperextension deformity at the metacarpophalangeal joints of the ring and little fingers and a flexion deformity of the other joints of these fingers. It is due to a loss of function, in particular of the interossei and the two lumbricals supplied by the ulnar nerve.

Dupuytren's contracture is due to a thickening of the palmar aponeurosis and of its extensions to the fingers. The ring and little fingers are predominantly affected. Thickened nodules are felt in the skin of the palm and there may be an associated flexion deformity of the metacarpophalangeal and proximal inter-phalangeal joints of the particular fingers.

Trigger finger is due to thickening of the flexor tendon and of its flexor sheath (Fig. 15.7). This thickening can be felt in line with the distal palmar crease. The finger will flex but extension is inhibited and may have to be done passively; when it occurs there is a painful click. In adults the ring and middle fingers are usually affected. In children the thumb is often involved.

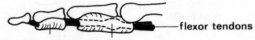

tunnels of fibrous flexor sheath   nodule — flexor tendons

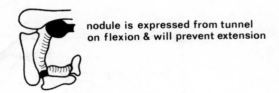

nodule is expressed from tunnel on flexion & will prevent extension

Fig. 15.7   Trigger finger.

Heberden's nodes are seen around the distal phalanges of fingers in patients with osteoarthritis.

Spindle swellings of the proximal interphalangeal joints are seen in patients who have rheumatoid arthritis.

Stability

The stability of each of the joints of the hand should be tested for integrity of the collateral ligaments.

Neurological examination

A brief neurological examination of the upper limb should be performed. Wasting should be observed over the thenar and hypothenar eminences and the interossei, in particular that of the first web space.

The motor power should be tested, in particular opposition of the thumb, function of the interossei, and the function of the flexor profundus of the little finger and the flexor profundus of the index finger.

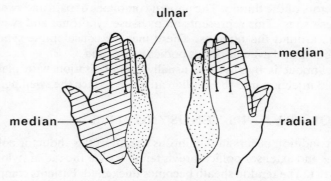

Fig. 15.8 Subcutaneous innervation of the hand.

Impairment of sensibility should be tested for touch and pain and two point discrimination over the median and ulnar nerve distributions in the hand (Fig. 15.8).

The neck and both upper limbs should be studied to complete the examination.

GANGLION

This is a cystic lesion which contains clear mucinous fluid. It is found most frequently over the dorsum of the wrist joint but may be found anywhere in the hand in relation to a joint or tendon sheath. Patients will complain of a swelling, sometimes painful.

The aetiology is unknown. It is probably a degenerative process; it sometimes occurs after trauma. Ganglia have a demonstrable fibrous connection to joint capsule or tendon sheath. However it is not possible to demonstrate communication between a synovial space and the contents of a ganglion.

Ganglia should only be excised if they are painful or causing symptoms from pressure on relating structures. If they are excised, there is a fair possibility of recurrence. They may be burst by pressure or aspirated but will almost inevitably recur after this sort of treatment.

TENOSYNOVITIS

A tenosynovitis occurs quite frequently around the extensor tendons of the fingers at the dorsum of the wrist and around the abductors of the thumb. The patient complains of pain and swelling at these sites. This represents an over-use syndrome and swelling occurs around the tendons. There may be considerable synovial thickening and even fibrinous bodies in the fluid.

Treatment is by rest and usually immobilisation with plaster. Steroid injection into the swollen area will reduce the swelling.

DE QUERVAIN'S TENOSYNOVITIS

This condition occurs in the fibrous sheath of the abductor pollicis longus and extensor pollicis brevis tendons over the radial styloid of the wrist. The tendon sheath becomes thickened. Patients complain of pain in the region of the radial styloid when using the wrist and on examination a tender nodule is found.

This can be managed conservatively by plaster and an injection of steroid into the tender nodule. However it is very effectively treated by a simple operation to split the tight tendon sheath.

TRIGGER FINGER (stenosing tenovaginitis)

This condition occurs frequently in middle-aged ladies as a painful nodule at the base of the middle or ring finger in the region of the distal palmar crease. The finger can usually be flexed fully but extension is painful and comes suddenly with a painful snap. The lesion consists of a thickening of the flexor tendon and of the flexor sheath at its proximal end (Fig. 15.7). The condition is sometimes associated with early rheumatoid arthritis.

TRIGGER THUMB

This is a similar lesion to the above, occurring in the flexor sheath of the flexor pollicis longus. The tendon nodule is in the region of the proximal skin crease at the base of the thumb. It is frequently seen in young children who will hold the thumb flexed and be unable to extend it. As a result, it may be confused with a contracture of the flexor pollicis longus or even a rupture of the extensor pollicis longus.

The most effective treatment is an operation to split the tight sheath of the flexor pollicis longus.

DUPUYTREN'S CONTRACTURE

This condition is frequently seen in middle-aged and elderly men. It is due to thickening of the palmar aponeurosis. The aponeurosis covers the centre of the palm and has extensions to each of the four fingers.

Initially the patients present with a nodule in the palm. This nodule is in the palmar fascia, and tends to be attached to the overlying skin. At a later stage, the thickened palmar fascia contracts. The contracture occurs firstly at the metacarpophalangeal joint and then at the proximal interphalangeal joint of the affected finger. The fingers involved are usually the little and ring fingers.

When the contracture starts developing, it is advisable to perform an operation to remove the affected palmar fascia. If neglected, the finger may contract to such an extent that the hand becomes useless. A severely contracted finger may warrant amputation. Removal of the contracted segment over the metacarpophalangeal joint will result in almost perfect correction. However if the proximal interphalangeal joint has been contracted for any length of time, the correction is liable to be incomplete. Before proceeding to operation, it is advisable to mention to the patient that one of the digital nerves of the finger may be damaged. The contracted tissue itself tends to infiltrate the web space between the fingers as an extension reaching down to the transverse metacarpal ligament. This extension may involve the digital nerve.

VOLKMANN'S CONTRACTURE

This is a very serious lesion which is unsatisfactory to treat. It follows the development of ischaemia and infarction in the flexor muscles of the forearm. The most common cause of this ischaemia is involvement of the brachial artery from a supracondylar fracture of the humerus or from a fracture or operation on the forearm bones. The brachial artery can be damaged either by direct involvement or secondary to a closed compartment syndrome in the forearm.

After the muscles become infarcted, they are replaced by fibrous tissue. This contracts and the patient is left with a severe contracture of the fingers and thumb.

The ischaemia involves not only the forearm muscles but also the median nerve and these patients have impaired function of the median nerve in the hand as well as the contracture.

Surgery is very difficult and the results are poor. In the majority of cases, this lesion is preventable and great care must be taken in the management of displaced supracondylar fractures and displaced fractures of the forearm.

CARPAL TUNNEL SYNDROME

This is a very common condition occurring classically in middle-aged ladies. The median nerve passes into the hand beneath the flexor retinaculum at the wrist, in company with the long flexor tendons to the fingers. Compression at this site can be caused by:

1. Hormonal conditions associated with water retention, such as pregnancy, menopause and contraceptives.

2. Trauma such as after a Colle's fracture.

3. Rheumatoid arthritis, probably due to involvement of the sheaths of the long flexor tendons to the fingers.

4. Rarely, space occupying lesions beneath the flexor retinaculum such as a ganglion or lipoma.

5. In many cases, no primary cause is found.

The patients complain of pain in the region of the wrist and fingers which is accompanied by numbness and tingling. These symptoms are worse at night and tend to wake the patient early in the morning. They may be relieved by altering the position of the hand.

On examination, there may be no definite physical signs. Occasionally pressure over the carpal tunnel will reproduce the symptoms. There may be wasting of the thenar eminence in severe cases. The neck is examined to exclude the cervical spine as a cause of the symptoms (it should be emphasised that cervical spondylosis and carpal tunnel syndrome can co-exist and relief of one may relieve the patient's symptoms).

Treatment may be conservative with diuretics and a night splint.

However the most effective treatment is a simple operation to release the flexor retinaculum at the wrist.

ULNAR NERVE COMPRESSION

The ulnar nerve can be compressed as it passes deep to the palm in close relation to the hook of the hamate. Pressure here will cause signs and symptoms in the distribution of the deep branch of the ulnar nerve. The patient will notice weakness of the hand and wasting of the intrinsic muscles particularly those of the first interspace. Such a lesion requires operative release.

MADELUNG'S DEFORMITY

This is a deformity of the wrist (Fig. 15.9) which usually occurs in girls. It is often bilateral and may be associated with a general osteochondrodystrophy. For some reason, growth is impaired at the lower radial epiphysis and, as a result, the ulnar styloid tends to become more prominent and subluxed dorsally and the radius may be bowed in a volar direction. The deformity is cosmetically not acceptable and also the patient may have lost some of the range of pronation and supination. In young children, a reasonable correction can be obtained by an osteotomy of the lower end of the radius. In older children, it is reasonable to excise the subluxed ulnar styloid.

A similar deformity can arise as a result of trauma, in particular fractures which damage the lower radial epiphyseal plate.

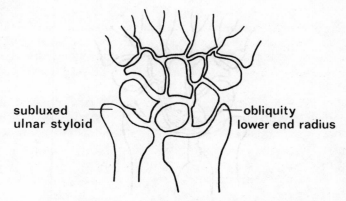

subluxed ulnar styloid — obliquity lower end radius

Fig. 15.9   Madelung's deformity; right wrist, palmar aspect.

RADIAL CLUB HAND

This is an uncommon condition which may be associated with multiple congenital deformities. The radius is attenuated and the thumb may be absent. As a result, the whole hand is deviated to the radial side on the forearm bones.

The deformity of the hand can be corrected by centralisation of the carpus on the ulna. If the thumb is absent, some function can be restored by pollicisation of the index finger. In some severe cases, the elbow joint is stiff or non-functional. In these cases the radial deviation of the hand is of benefit to the patient as he can reach his mouth by means of shoulder movements. In such patients, no operative correction should be attempted.

OSTEOCHONDROSIS OF THE LUNATE
(Kienbock's disease)

In this condition, the lunate shows avascular changes (Fig. 15.10). These may result from an actual dislocation or from repeated minor trauma. It occurs usually in active young men, who complain of persistent aching pain of the wrist on activity and possibly an associated swelling. If the symptoms are persistent and are interfering with the patient's activities, it is reasonable to replace the lunate with a Silastic prosthesis. If the condition has progressed to the extent of generalised degenerative changes in the wrist, a wrist arthrodesis may be necessary.

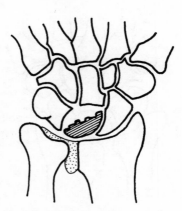

Fig. 15.10   Kienbock's disease: avascular necrosis of lunate.

OSTEOARTHRITIS OF THE WRIST

Osteoarthritis of the wrist occurs usually as a result of trauma or as a result of avascular necrosis of the lunate or proximal pole of the scaphoid (Fig. 15.11). Patients will complain of pain and swelling around the wrist and on examination, movements will be limited. X-rays will show characteristic changes.

1st metacarpal / trapezium joint

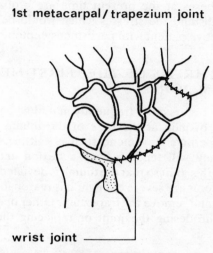

wrist joint

Fig. 15.11   Osteoarthritis of the wrist.

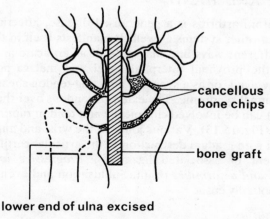

cancellous bone chips

bone graft

lower end of ulna excised

Fig. 15.12   Arthrodesis of the wrist.

In many patients, reduction of activities involving the wrist and the use of a splint may be adequate to control the symptoms. However, if the patient requires a strong forearm and hand, there is no alternative to arthrodesis of the wrist (Fig. 15.12). Patients with an arthrodesed wrist will have no pain and will have practically full range of pronation and supination. There will of course be no movement actually in the wrist joint.

Wrist prostheses at the present time are probably not strong enough to withstand the stresses which would be imposed upon them by the active patient with persistent symptoms.

OSTEOARTHRITIS OF THE FIRST METACARPAL TRAPEZIUM JOINT

This condition occurs quite frequently in middle-aged ladies. They will complain of pain at the base of the thumb particularly on performing repetitive movements such as knitting. If the condition progresses, they will tend to have a flexion and an adduction contracture at this joint so that the thumb is deviated into the palm.

If the symptoms are severe enough, it is reasonable to operate on these patients and remove the trapezium. Other operations devised consist of arthrodesing the joint or replacing the trapezium by Silastic prosthesis.

RHEUMATOID ARTHRITIS AFFECTING THE WRIST AND HAND

Rheumatoid arthritis is a generalised disease, affecting not only joints but other systems as well. It manifests itself in the hands in many different ways and may present as an acute arthritis, with mainly the proximal interphalangeal and metacarpophalangeal joints involved, or as a synovitis affecting tendon sheaths, causing carpal tunnel syndrome. The extensor tendons over the dorsum of the wrist can be involved chronically and tendon ruptures occur at this site (Fig. 15.13). Various joints of the wrist and fingers may be involved with gradual destruction of the articular cartilage and the attachment of associated ligaments. *Progressive loss of joint function and deformities* result. Subluxation and even dislocation may eventually ensue.

Acute arthritis
Acute arthritis is seen in the proximal interphalangeal joints where

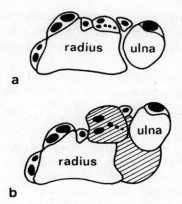

Fig. 15.13 Extensor compartments of left wrist, pronated; (a) normal, (b) extensor communis tendons infiltrated by rheumatoid-synovium.

it causes a spindle type swelling of the fingers. At this stage, the treatment is essentially conservative with drugs and rest. Physiotherapy to restore movements is important in the convalescent stage. An acute arthritis can involve the metacarpophalangeal joint and cause an acutely painful swelling here. If these joints are to be splinted, they should be splinted at 90° flexion.

Chronic arthritis
The metacarpophalangeal joints may be the site of persistent swelling from thickened synovium. At this stage, a chemical synovectomy may be of value; intra-articular steroids are frequently used.

As the condition progresses, the capsule of the metacarpophalangeal joint is stretched and the extensor tendons shift medially. As a result, a classical ulnar deviation deformity develops at these joints. This is unpleasing cosmetically but the function of the metacarpophalangeal joints and of the fingers remains reasonably satisfactory as long as a good range of movements is retained. In order to prevent an ulnar deviation deformity progressing, an operative synovectomy may be performed on the metacarpophalangeal joints.

However, the metacarpals may actually sublux or dislocate and in these cases function can be partly restored by inserting Silastic prostheses and reefing the joint capsule so that the fingers are realigned. It must be remembered that there is usually no increase in range of movements at the metacarpophalangeal joints after this procedure.

The disease may progress at the proximal interphalangeal joints, and cause damage to the ligamentous attachments, particularly that of the volar plate. Similarly, the insertion of the sublimis tendon into the middle phalanx may be eroded. Deformities can occur at the proximal interphalangeal joint and one of the most common is the *swan neck deformity* with hyperextension at the proximal interphalangeal joint with associated flexion at the distal interphalangeal joint. This deformity is accentuated by a contracture of the intrinsic muscles as they are inserted into the extensor expansion. A satisfactory surgical correction of this deformity is difficult to obtain.

All joints of the thumb may be involved – that between the first metacarpal and the trapezium, the first metacarpophalangeal joint and the distal interphalangeal joint. Diseases of these joints cause an *adduction contracture of the thumb*, which deviates into the palm. At the first metacarpophalangeal joint, the ligaments may be slackened, and the joint becomes unstable and tends to sublux very easily. Surgical treatment is confined to stabilisation of the joints and release of the adduction contractures.

The *wrist joint* itself is frequently involved in rheumatoid arthritis. There is frequently boggy synovial proliferation which is difficult to resolve. This may be accompanied by subluxation dorsally of the ulnar styloid. In association with this, there may be proliferated thickened synovium around the *extensor tendons* (Fig. 15.13) which can be removed by a synovectomy to improve function. The ulnar styloid can also be excised. If any of the extensor tendons have been ruptured, they can be repaired by a tendon transfer.

If the wrist joint is very badly damaged, an arthrodesis will stabilise it. A prosthesis for the wrist joint has recently been described, but it is not yet certain how useful it will be.

CHAPTER 16

Elbow Joint and Shoulder

ELBOW

History taking

Pain, which is often well localised, is the commonest complaint of patients with elbow lesions. Stiffness may be a symptom and in particular patients may complain of locking (a mechanical block to movement). There may be deformity.

There may be tingling or other peripheral nerve symptoms, in particular in the distribution of the ulnar nerve.

Any history of injury should be determined.

Examination

This is done with the patient standing or sitting. Both elbows should be examined simultaneously. It is best to have the patient strip to the waist and have both upper limbs fully exposed.

Inspection

Bony and soft tissue contours are examined (Fig. 16.1), and any deformities of valgus or varus which occur at the elbow are noted (Fig. 16.2). Any particular swellings are noted; an effusion of the elbow may be seen in the olecranon fossa or adjacent to the radial head. Any scars or other lesions are noted.

Palpation

Tender areas are palpated, particularly over the epicondyles.

The bony contours are palpated (note that there is an equilateral triangle formed by both epicondyles and the tip of the olecranon

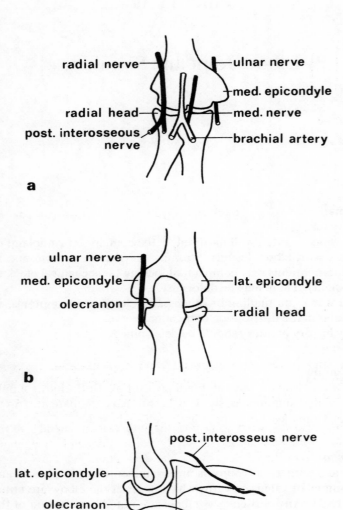

Fig. 16.1   Aspects of elbow (a) anterior, (b) posterior, (c) landmarks
of lateral side

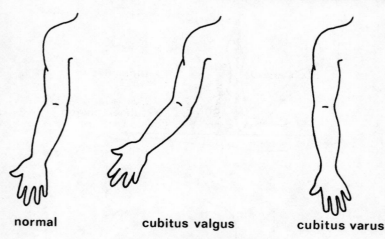

normal   cubitus valgus   cubitus varus

Fig. 16.2 Deformities of elbow.

which can be used to demonstrate normal contours around the elbow).

Soft tissue contours are also palpated. The peripheral pulses are felt. Temperature of the joint is noted.

Movements

Active and passive movements should be measured. Flexion–extension range is from 0° in full extension to about 150° full flexion when the forearm comes in contact with the muscles of the upper limb (Fig. 16.3). Rotation movements involve not only the elbow joint but also the wrist joint and the interosseous membrane in between. The arm should be held to the side with the elbow touching the side of the body and pronation and supination estimated. There is a 180° range of pronation–supination.

The stability of the elbow to both valgus and varus stresses should be determined.

Neurological examination

Neurological examination of the hand, in particular of the ulnar nerve, should be performed. Any wasting of the intrinsic muscles of the hand should be noted and sensation tested.

To complete the examination the neck and the rest of the upper limb are examined.

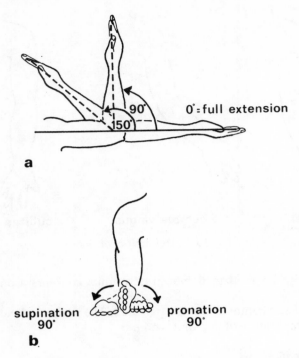

Fig. 16.3 Measuring elbow movements; (a) elbow flexion, (b) forearm rotation.

Lesions about the elbow joint

'Tennis elbow' — lateral epicondylitis (Fig. 16.4)

This is a very common syndrome. The patients complain of pain in the region of the lateral epicondyle which is made worse by any strenuous use of the forearm or hand. On examination, there is tenderness, over the lateral epicondyle. Stressing the common extensor origin by resisted extension of the wrist produces pain.

The symptoms often follow persistent over-use of the elbow, and is therefore frequent in tennis and squash players. It may also be found after a direct knock on the elbow, with the symptoms persisting.

Treatment involves primarily rest. An injection of local anaesthetic and steroids often has dramatic effects. The symptoms may be persistent and chronic. Patients may be relieved by repeated

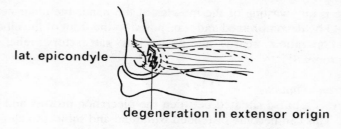

lat. epicondyle

degeneration in extensor origin

Fig. 16.4   Tennis elbow.

injections or by immobilising the elbow in plaster. In some cases, operation is advised and various procedures are described to relieve symptoms. The variety of procedures is evidence of their effectiveness. Patients with persistent symptoms should have a serum uric acid test performed to exclude gouty diathesis.

Medial epicondylitis (golfer's elbow)
This lesion affects the medial epicondyle. Fortunately it resolves easily with rest. Steroid injections into this site should only be given with caution as the ulnar nerve is in close proximity.

Ulnar nerve neuritis
The ulnar nerve runs through a fibro-osseous tunnel behind the medial epicondyle of the elbow. The nerve is liable to be compressed in this tunnel if there are any projecting osteophytes. If the elbow has a valgus deformity, the ulnar nerve is liable to be stretched as it goes through the tunnel.

Patients will complain of pain in the region of the medial epicondyle. They will have symptoms of numbness and tingling in the course of the ulnar nerve which will be felt primarily over the ring and little fingers and the ulnar side of the palm of the hand. There may be a feeling of weakness in the forearm and hand.

Transient ulnar nerve neuritis may occur after a contusion or be found in patients using elbow crutches.

On examination, there may be wasting of the small muscles of the hand (particularly seen in the first web space). There will also be impairment of sensation over the ulnar nerve distribution of the hand. Tapping of the ulnar nerve at the medial epicondyle will produce a positive Tinel sign.

However, if the symptoms are persistent, and in particular if there is any wasting of the muscles of the hand, the ulnar nerve should be decompressed and transposed to the front of the elbow. This operation nearly always affords satisfactory relief of symptoms.

Olecranon bursitis

There is a bursa situated between the olecranon process and the skin. This can become distended with fluid and subject to chronic inflammation. The patient will present with a fluctuant swollen bursa which may be subject to infection.

If the symptoms are persistent, the fluid should be aspirated and a compression bandage applied. Operative removal of this lesion is frequently followed by delayed healing and should only be performed if there is no alternative.

This region of the elbow is a common site for rheumatoid nodules and a patient with rheumatoid arthritis may have olecranon bursitis as well. The nodules require removal only if the patient has very significant symptoms.

Lesions of the elbow joint

Loose bodies

Loose bodies occur in the elbow joint and these can give rise to symptoms of pain and swelling and also of locking. The 'locking' will cause the elbow to jam in one position and may cause considerable distress.

The commonest cause of loose bodies in the elbow joint are:
Osteochondritis disseccans, usually of the capitellum.
As a result of fracture (such as of the radial head).
Following arthritis about the elbow.

If the loose bodies are causing significant symptoms they should be removed.

Osteochondritis disseccans

This lesion occurs around the elbow joint in the region of the capitellum. It is frequently bilateral. The fragment may be shed into the joint causing symptoms of a loose body.

Osteoarthritis in the elbow

This condition is not uncommonly found in the elbow joint. It occurs more frequently after trauma. The elbow is not a weight-bearing joint and a patient suffering from symptoms of osteoarthritis around the elbow can usually be helped with advice about activities. It is only rarely that operative treatment is required which is fortunate as elbow prostheses are at present unsatisfactory. Arthrodesis of the elbow is probably the most effective operation.

Rheumatoid arthritis

When this occurs in the region of the elbow it is usually a sign of widespread disease involving many joints. There may be considerable synovial thickening about the elbow and this may protrude through the capsule, causing swelling. The capsule may be stretched and permit the radial head to sublux. The condition can usually be managed by conservative treatment by steroid injections and immobilisation in the acute stage. However, if the symptoms persist and the radial head subluxation causes significant pain, it is reasonable to perform a synovectomy of the elbow joint including excision of the radial head. The prostheses for elbow replacement are not satisfactory at the present time. An arthrodesis of the elbow should rarely be performed in patients with rheumatoid arthritis as so many other joints are involved.

THE SHOULDER

History taking

Pain

Pain is the predominant complaint of patients with shoulder lesions. It may be felt in the region of the shoulder and the radiation is classically to the upper arm as far as, but not distal to, the elbow.

Stiffness

Stiffness is frequently complained of in association with pain and occasionally without pain.

Patients will complain of difficulty with using their arms above shoulder level. They complain frequently of pain on dressing and doing their hair.

History of injury

In adults the majority of painful shoulder lesions are due to degenerative changes of the rotator cuff. Symptoms may be noted after injury but the trauma is usualy trifling.

Neck lesions
Shoulder lesions are frequently associated with neck lesions, such as cervical spondylosis.

Related disease
Such diseases include coronary occlusions, stroke, gall bladder disease, hiatus hernia and others.

Examination
Movements of the shoulder occur not only at the gleno-humeral joint but also at the joint between the scapula and the chest wall. During normal shoulder action, movement occurs at both joints simultaneously. It is essential to examine both shoulders, comparing them throughout the examination. The patient is required to strip to the waist so that the neck and upper limbs can be seen as well as the shoulder.

Inspection (Fig. 16.5)
Inspection should be from above, then from behind, then from in front. One looks for any deformity, for abnormalities of contour or wasting, particularly of the deltoid muscle, and for any scars or other lesion.

Palpation
Palpate for local tenderness over the coracoid, the subacromial bursa, and the biceps tendon. Bony contours, which include the clavicle, acromion, spine of scapula, and head of the humerus (which is felt anterior to the acromion), and soft tissue contours of the muscles concerned, must be palpated. The contents of the axilla should be palpated.

Measurement
The girth of the upper limb at the site of maximum diameter should be measured. Note that the dominant arm usually has 1 cm greater girth than the other arm.

Active and passive movements
The movements tested are abduction, flexion, internal and external rotation (Fig. 16.6). Abduction movement occurs in the coronal plane, flexion and extension movement in the sagittal.

The range of movements is measured and the results expressed in

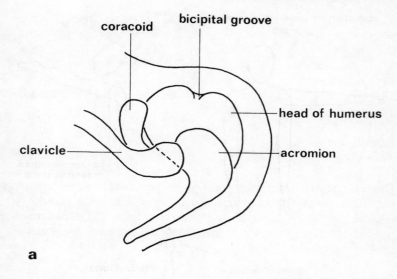

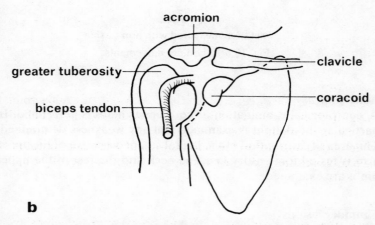

Fig. 16.5   Shoulder landmarks from (a) above, and (b) in front.

degrees. Any pain on performing these movements is noted. A syndrome called the painful arc syndrome is described where the first 60° of abduction are pain-free and then the patient will complain of pain until about 120°. Such a painful arc of abduction is found in patients who have a rotator cuff lesion (Fig. 16.7).

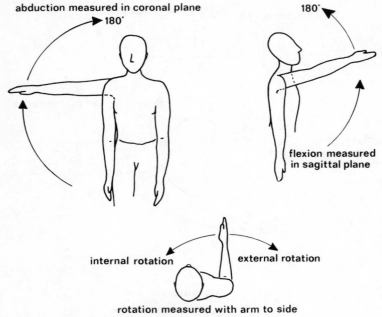

abduction measured in coronal plane
180°

180°

flexion measured
in sagittal plane

internal rotation   external rotation

rotation measured with arm to side

Fig. 16.6   Shoulder movements.

Neurological

A neurological examination of both upper limbs is performed. In particular the deltoid is examined and any weakness determined. The area of distribution of the lateral cutaneous nerve of the upper arm is tested for sensory loss. The neck and the rest of the upper limbs are examined.

Shoulder lesions

Recurrent dislocation of the shoulder

The shoulder nearly always dislocates anteriorly and inferiorly. The lesion occurs as a result of injury in young people. As a result of injury, the capsule of the shoulder joint is stretched and sometimes the glenoid labrum is detached. If healing does not occur, the shoulder is liable to recurrences of dislocation.

The patient is usualy a young fit male, who gives a history of initial dislocation and of two or three subsequent dislocations. The

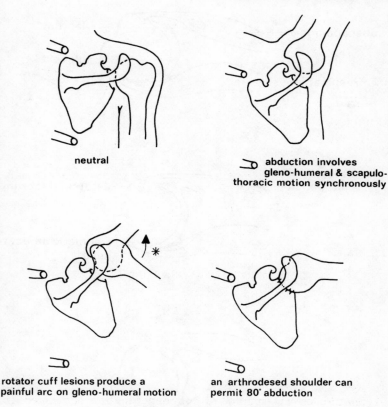

neutral

abduction involves
gleno-humeral & scapulo-
thoracic motion synchronously

rotator cuff lesions produce a
painful arc on gleno-humeral motion

an arthrodesed shoulder can
permit 80° abduction

Fig. 16.7 Shoulder movements.

shoulder will usually dislocate with a combination of abduction and
external rotation movements at the gleno-humeral joint. The
symptoms are quite distressing and the only effective treatment is
by operation. The most commonly performed operation is the
Putti-Platt operation. In this, the anterior pouch of the capsule is
obliterated and the capsule and the overlying subscapularis tendon
are tightened as much as possible (Fig. 16.8).

The condition also occurs in patients who have congenital laxity
of joints. This type is found more frequently in young ladies. They
are found to have hyper-mobile joints and exhibit excessive
extension of the metacarpophalangeal joints of the fingers, the
elbows and the knees. Their shoulders tend to dislocate easily.

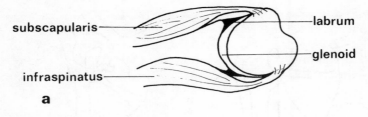

subscapularis—

—labrum

—glenoid

infraspinatus—

a

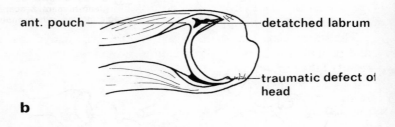

ant. pouch—

—detatched labrum

—traumatic defect of head

b

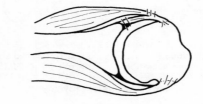

c

Fig. 16.8 (a) Normal shoulder, (b) pathology after recurrent dislocation, (c) Putti-Platt repair.

These patients will not receive adequate benefit from operation, and should be advised to restrict activities so the shoulder does not dislocate.

The acromio-clavicular joint
The acromio-clavicular joint may dislocate after a fall on the point of the shoulder. This dislocation is accompanied by a rupture of the coraco-clavicular ligament.

Patients may present with a long standing dislocation of the acromio-clavicular joint. On examination, they will have a prominence of the clavicle above the acromion on the point of the shoulder. In most patients, there are only minimal symptoms and no active treatment is required. However, if it is painful the outer end of the clavicle can be excised.

The sterno-clavicular joint

The sterno-clavicular joint can also dislocate. In some patients, recurrent dislocation of this joint occurs. They will complain of a painful clicking in the region of a manubrium sterni as the end of the clavicle dislocates. This recurrent dislocation can be cured by operation, if the symptoms warrant it.

The sterno-clavicular joint is also subject to rheumatoid arthritis and patients can present with a painful swelling of this joint as a result of the process.

Rotator cuff lesions

On moving the arm from the side, movement occurs between the scapula and chest wall and between the humerus and the scapula at the gleno-humeral joint.

The stability of the gleno-humeral joint depends very largely on the tendons of the adjacent muscles. The tendons of these muscles are very closely related indeed to the capsule of the gleno-humeral joint. These tendons are known as the rotator cuff and include the subscapularis in front, the supraspinatus above and the infraspinatus and teres minor behind (Fig. 16.9).

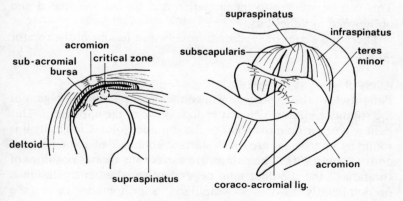

Fig. 16.9   Rotator cuff.

The blood supply of these tendons is rather tenuous and can easily be interrupted. The tendons are then liable to degenerative change. As a result of this degenerative change, a partial rupture is frequent and complete ruptures occasionally occur. In addition in the areas of degeneration, deposits of calcium are sometimes found and may cause symptoms (Fig. 16.10).

The symptoms from these changes are accentuated by degenerative changes in the acromio-clavicular joint.

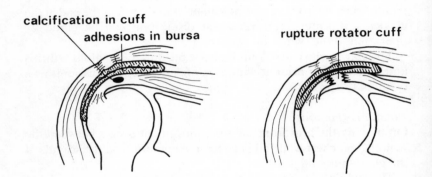

Fig. 16.10   Rotator cuff lesions.

Sometimes the long head of biceps is involved as it passes through the rotator cuff direct to its attachment on the superior aspect of the glenoid.

Between the rotator cuff and the deltoid is the subacromial bursa. This can be subject to inflammation and become thickened and obliterated by adhesions.

There is a series of syndromes ascribed to lesions of the rotator cuff.

PAINFUL ARC SYNDROME
Patients with this syndrome will complain of pain in the region of the shoulder joint, which may radiate down to the upper arm. This pain will occur on movement of the shoulder joint. Classically it is found as a particular arc which starts at about 60° of abduction and ends at about 120°. The painful arc varies with various positions of rotation of the shoulder joint depending on whether the lesion is predominantly in the subscapularis, supraspinatus or in the posterior tendons (see Fig. 16.7).

X-ray may show evidence of calcium in the tendons around the shoulder. There is frequently sclerosis in the greater tuberosity of the humerus at the attachment of the supraspinatus tendon. There may be associated degenerative changes in the acromio-clavicular joint.

These symptoms usually occur in the middle-aged person. They may occur spontaneously but often appear after a minor injury. They are very resistant to treatment.

Treatment is essentially conservative and includes:

Judicious use of analgesic and anti-inflammatory tablets.

The injection of local anaesthetic and steroid into the subacromial bursa.

When the acute stage has subsided, graduated exercises with a physiotherapist are required. She may prescribe various other remedies.

Occasionally the symptoms are persistent and sufficiently distressing to warrant operation. One of the commonly performed operations involves excision of the coraco-acromial ligament and the anterior portion of the acromion. This relieves the pressure on the rotator cuff. If the acromio-clavicular joint is involved, the outer end of the clavicle is also excised.

COMPLETE RUPTURE

Complete rupture of the rotator cuff occasionally occurs. This is usually as a result of a fall or sudden jolt in an elderly patient. The patient will present with inability to lift the arm from the side. There may not be any severe pain. The passive movements are usually full range.

In these elderly patients, the best treatment is conservative and in due course the patient will be able to use his arm adequately. Operation to repair the rotator cuff is difficult and the results tend to be disappointing.

ACUTE CALCIFICATION SYNDROME

Occasionally young ladies will present with severe pain in the shoulder. This pain is so severe that it will interfere with sleep and prevent any movement of the shoulder. X-ray will show calcification in the region of the rotator cuff.

The calcification in these patients appears to set up an acute inflammatory reaction in the tendons of the rotator cuff. The symptoms can sometimes be relieved by aspiration which will permit the calcium to escape from the confines of the rotator cuff. If this fails, a small open operation will give relief of the acute symptoms.

FROZEN SHOULDER SYNDROME
In some patients, symptoms of the painful arc syndrome may progress to those of the frozen shoulder syndrome. Patients involved usually have suffered a severe illness such as a coronary thrombosis. They complain of severe pain in the shoulder region and in the upper arm. They find that the shoulder is too painful to move and on examination the passive range of movements in the shoulder is grossly limited. X-ray may show signs similar to that of the painful arc syndrome. Initially this lesion should be managed conservatively much on the lines of the painful arc syndrome. After two or three months it is reasonable to inject the subacromial bursa and gently manipulate the shoulder under an anaesthetic. This may be accompanied by dramatic relief of symptoms. In some patients the pain gradually resolves itself and the patient is left with a stiff gleno-humeral joint. However he will be left with about 80° range of abduction and flexion which will be sufficient for ordinary purposes. This movement will occur between the scapula and the chest wall.

Bicipital tendonitis
Sometimes the patient's symptoms are confined to the area of the long head of the biceps in the region of the shoulder. In these cases, the term bicipital tendinitis is used to describe the lesion. The treatment is much as described for the painful arc syndrome.

Rupture of the long head of the biceps
In middle aged or elderly men the long head of the biceps is quite likely to rupture as a result of sudden exertion. They will present with a swelling of the biceps in the upper arm. There is usually no treatment required unless they are complaining of continual pain and clicking in the shoulder. In such patients, exploration of the shoulder can be performed to remove the proximal end of the biceps tendon.

Rheumatoid arthritis in the shoulder region
Patients with rheumatoid arthritis may present with a painful arc syndrome or with a frozen shoulder.
     Long-standing rheumatoid arthritis can cause persistent pain and

severe limitation of movement in the gleno-humeral joint. X-rays will show gross narrowing of the joint space and sometimes necrotic changes in the head of the humerus.

This syndrome is very difficult to treat as these patients have very distressing and severe symptoms. Ideally, the shoulder should be arthrodesed but technically this is a very difficult operation demanding a long period of immobilisation in a body plaster. Patients who would benefit from this operation are not able to withstand the period of immobilisation. Similar changes in the shoulder joint are also seen in old people, particularly those who have had a frozen shoulder for any length of time. They also have a most distressing stiff and painful shoulder and the treatment is very unsatisfactory.

Various prostheses have been devised to replace the shoulder joint. However, none of these is at present in general use.

CHAPTER 17

The Neck

HISTORY TAKING

Pain

Pain is the predominant symptom of patients with neck lesions; the following should be noted:

Site. It is usually necessary to get the patient to point to the site of the pain.

Duration of symptoms and whether persistent or episodic.

Predisposing and relieving factors.

History of injury. It is important to find out how closely symptoms are related to an injury.

Radiation to occiput, across 'shoulders', to dorsal spine and down arms to fingers of hands. The patient should point out the extent of the pain.

Previous treatment, and how effective it has been.

Feeling of instability. A feeling of 'head falling off' occurs with patients with an unstable cervical spine and should be taken seriously.

Upper limb symptoms of weakness, numbness and paraesthesiae.

Lower limb symptoms of weakness and clumsiness may indicate long-tract involvement.

Visceral symptoms are ascribed by some to neck conditions. Lesions of throat, pharynx, oesophagus and other cervical viscera should be considered.

Examination

The patient should strip to the waist and be examined standing or sitting. Examine (from in front and from behind).

140

Inspect:

    Deformities such as torticollis or webbing.

    Level of shoulders.

    Dorsal spine for kyphosis or lordosis.

Palpate:

    Spines and disc spaces.

    For local tenderness over spines posteriorly, over posterior triangle, over brachial plexus, and either side of trachea in front of neck.

    Soft tissues of neck.

Movements:

    Flexion and extension.

    Rotation.

    Lateral flexion (often very limited in elderly people).

Neurological examination of upper limbs

    Test for biceps, triceps, brachioradialis reflexes.

    Test muscle power of main groups of muscles.

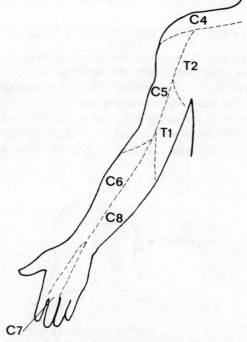

Fig. 17.1   Dermatomes in the upper limb.

Measure upper arm and forearms for wasting.

Test sensory loss over dermatomes in upper limbs (Fig. 17.1).

Examine all joints of the upper limbs especially the shoulders and examine dorsal and lumbar spine.

Examine mouth and throat.

In some cases a neurological examination of the lower limbs is indicated, in particular for loss of proprioception, weakness and spasticity.

X-rays of the cervical spine should include:

Routine AP and lateral views involving all cervical vertebrae and to exclude a cervical rib.

Flexion and extension lateral views of the cervical spine to demonstrate segmental instability.

Through-mouth views to show the atlas and odontoid.

Oblique views to show intervertebral foramina.

A myelogram is sometimes of value to localise a lesion or exclude a neoplasm.

CONGENITAL TORTICOLLIS (Fig. 17.2)

This condition occurs in infants and in young children. It probably develops just after birth when the first sign is that of a 'sterno-mastoid tumour'. In due course, the sterno-mastoid appears to contract and the head is tilted on one side.

The patient with torticollis will present with a permanently tilted head. The sterno-mastoid is felt as a thick fibrous contracted cord. There may be facial asymmetry. There is no underlying bone abnormality.

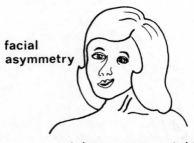

facial
asymmetry

tight sterno-mastoid

Fig. 17.2   Torticollis.

If the lesion is seen early, it can be treated by manipulation. However, frequently it is best managed by an open operation to divide the tight sterno-mastoid. Physiotherapy should be continued afterwards. If the lesion is allowed to persist, a very definite facial asymmetry will develop, and the patient will hold the head on one side even though the contracture has been released.

ABNORMALITIES OF THE CERVICAL VERTEBRAE

There is a condition of congenital fusion of the cervical vertebrae known as the Klippel-Feil syndrome (Fig. 17.3). These people have short necks and a low hairline. It may be associated with a high

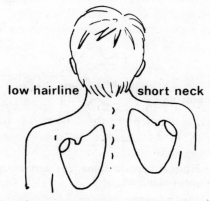

Fig. 17.3   Congenital high scapula (Sprengl's shoulder).

scapula (Sprengl's shoulder). These patients may develop a high scoliosis. There may also be atrophy of the upper limb on the affected side.

CERVICAL SPONDYLOSIS (Fig. 17.4b)

Degenerative changes in the discs of the cervical spine occur normally. Sometimes these changes are accelerated at certain levels and are reflected in X-ray abnormalities of the cervical spine. These X-ray abnormalities include:
  1. Narrowing of the disc space concerned.

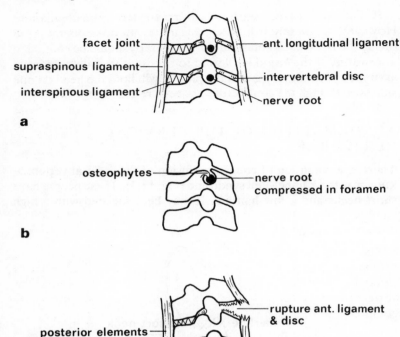

Fig. 17.4 (a) Normal cervical spine, (b) cervical spondylosis, (c) hypertension injury (whiplash).

2. Osteophyte formation at this level which tends to intrude into the intervertebral foramen as well as the vertebral canal.

3. Degenerative changes at the inter-facet joints of the cervical spine.

It is possible that injury can predispose the spine to these changes. The majority of patients with these X-ray changes can remember no significant injury to account for them, and frequently have no symptoms.

However, some patients do present with significant symptoms in their necks and arms and in association have the X-ray changes of cervical spondylosis. These patients complain of symptoms as follows:

1. Pain in the neck, which may be very severe. This may radiate to the occiput, across the shoulders, to the dorsal spine, and down one arm.

2. Stiffness in the neck. Associated with this may be sensations of clicking or creaking. This stiffness is noted particularly in playing sports and in performing such functions as reversing of a car.

3. There may be a great many associated symptoms such as numbness or tingling in the arms, weakness of the arm or hand, loss of sensation in the arm or hand, headaches (which are traditionally occipital but may radiate to the frontal region), feeling of dizziness or nausea.

4. Significant severe symptoms include weakness or clumsiness of the lower limbs (this may be related to cervical cord compression), and so-called 'drop attacks'. This is a rare but well documented phenomenon due to occlusion of the vertebral artery.

The symptoms of cervical spondylosis are mainly due to the osteophytic protrusions which involve the nerve root as it passes through the intervertebral foramen. They may also narrow the vertebral canal and compress the spinal cord. Sometimes they may compress the vertebral artery as it passes through its foramina.

Treatment
These patients are subject to exacerbations and remissions of symptoms. The treatment therefore is conservative and includes:

1. Immobilisation with collar during severe symptoms. This may be soft rubber collar or a firm plastic collar.

2. The neck can be controlled firmly at night by use of a 'butterfly' pillow or the patient can be instructed to wear his collar at night. Further neck protection can be given by using head rests in the car and sitting in a comfortable arm chair. Advice should be given on occupations which involve sitting with the head forward such as typing and sewing.

3. Analgesic and anti-inflammatory tablets can be prescribed.

4. Physiotherapy may cause an alleviation of the acute symptoms.

Surgery is rarely indicated. Indications are:

1. Disease localised to one single area causing intractible symptoms. This type of lesion is suitable for an anterior (dowel type) cervical fusion.

2. Patients with long-tract signs in the lower limbs can be treated

by a decompression laminectomy. The results are often disappointing. Furthermore, this operation tends to lead to some instability of the cervical spine and should always be accompanied by a posterior fusion.

'WHIP LASH' INJURIES OF THE CERVICAL SPINE (Fig. 17.4c)

Among the mechanisms of cervical spine injury has been described a hyperextension injury of the cervical spine. In this injury, the anterior longitudinal ligament, then the disc, and then the posterior longitudinal ligament at the back of the vertebral bodies, are successively ruptured. If healing is not permitted to occur, then this segment of the cervical spine will be unstable and jerking movements will cause pain. It is possible, as a result of such an injury, for disc material to be dislodged posteriorly on either side of the longitudinal ligament causing impingement of the root at that level. Such impingement may cause significant and objective neurological signs in the upper limbs, in the distribution of the nerve root affected.

This hyperextension injury can result from a road traffic accident, in particular the so-called 'shunt' accident where a car has been hit from behind causing the driver's head to flex forward towards the windscreen and then whiplash back over the seat of the car.

The patient with a significant and genuine whiplash injury will complain of pain in the neck a few hours after the accident. On examination, there will be tenderness over the anterior aspect of the neck. All movements will be limited. There may be objective neurological signs in the upper limbs such as loss of reflex in the area affected.

These patients are best managed with rest in bed and immobilisation of the neck with a firm collar. Analgesic tablets and tranquilisers should be prescribed. After about four weeks of such treatment, gentle physiotherapy should be instituted. Most cases will then resolve conservatively.

Operative treatment is only indicated in this condition if the level affected can be precisely localised. If so, dramatic relief of symptoms can be achieved by an anterior cervical fusion.

It should be emphasised that the majority of patients complaining of whiplash syndrome do not fill the above criteria, and do not demonstrate any objective disability as the result of such an accident.

CERVICAL DISC LESIONS

It is possible for the degenerative cervical disc to protrude in the manner of a lumbar disc. These patients will complain of pain in the neck and usually have symptoms radiating down the arm as the disc material impinges on the affected nerve root. This lesion is not nearly as common as that in the lumbar region.

In the majority of patients, the symptoms will resolve with conservative management as outlined above. If conservative management fails and the site of the lesion can be precisely localised, the symptoms can be dramatically relieved by an anterior cervical fusion. However, it should be stated that in most patients with these symptoms, the lesion cannot be precisely localised.

CHAPTER 18

Dorsal and Lumbar Spine

Back pain is a very common symptom. It may be caused by a variety of conditions which can be diagnosed precisely as significant lesions. However a great many cases are not diagnosable and treatment of these remains symptomatic.

Even if a spinal abnormality is discovered, it may well not be the only cause of the patient's symptoms. Furthermore, all patients who complain of back pain have some degree of functional overlay. In some it is minimal, but in many it adds significantly to the complaint. Assessment of the severity of back pain is difficult. Patients may have back pain which does not arise from the vertebral column but from some other system. These patients nearly always have symptoms related to that other system.

HISTORY TAKING

The site of pain
Patients cannot tell you precisely where it hurts. It is necessary therefore to ask them to point to the site of the pain.

Radiation of pain
Pain from the dorsal spine may radiate in 'girdle' fashion around the trunk along the line of the intercostal nerves. Pain from the upper dorsal spine tends to radiate to the neck and 'across the shoulder blades'. Pain from the lower dorsal spine can be felt in the lumbar region. It may be useful to have an X-ray of the dorsal spine when investigating patients with low back pain.

Pain from the upper lumbar spine can radiate to the front of the thighs and knees (mimicking hip pain). Pain from the lower lumbar spine can radiate to the coccyx, the buttocks and the greater trochanter. It can be felt as sciatica down the backs of the lower limbs to the heel and to the foot.

Exacerbating factors
These include standing, heavy lifting and twisting movements. Pain exacerbated by coughing or sneezing is associated with an intraspinal lesion such as a disc protrusion.

Relieving factors
These factors include bed rest, analgesics and other forms of treatment. In particular it should be noted if pain is *not* relieved by bed rest or if the patient is kept awake at night by back pain. Patients with such pain may have a very significant lesion such as infection or a tumour.

Severity of pain
This can be assessed by determining how much the patient is restricted by back pain. The patient should be asked what he cannot do because of the pain in his back. Patients with really severe back pain have to lie flat in bed. It is very difficult to determine how severe the pain is, since people with back pain often have a considerable functional overlay.

However, patients with very severe back conditions such as tumour or an infection may have such severe pain that they behave quite irrationally and unfortunately in consequence are liable to be labelled as 'functional'. Patients with back pain who behave irrationally require very careful assessment indeed.

Associated symptoms
These include symptoms such as numbness and tingling in the lower limb. Such symptoms are often related to nerve root lesions. Patients with back pain due to a visceral or cardiovascular cause will often complain of symptoms related to these systems as well as complaining of their back pain.

Duration of symptoms
It should be noted whether the pain is present continuously or intermittently. The length of, predisposition to, and relief of, each episode should be noted. Patients who have had symptoms for

twenty years need different treatment than those who have had symptoms for a week or two.

Previous treatment
It is essential to determine any previous treatment the patient may have had.

EXAMINATION

The patient should be stripped to his underwear. He should be examined standing, lying supine and then lying prone (Fig. 18.1).

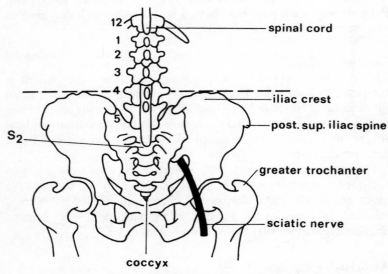

Fig. 18.1   Bony landmarks of lumbar spine, pelvis and hip.

Examination with the patient standing
Inspection for postural abnormalities and deformities. A lateral curvature can be a list or a scoliosis.

A *list* is a pure sideways curve of the spine and may be purely postural, as associated with a short leg on one side, or it may be due to muscle spasm as produced by nerve root irritation from a disc lesion. When the patient bends forwards a postural list is 'ironed out'. That due to muscle spasm tends to be accentuated but there is no evidence of rotation of the spine (Fig. 18.2).

Scoliosis is a lateral curve associated with rotation. This is a structural lesion. If the patient is observed standing, the shoulders may be uneven or the pelvis may show obliquity. If the patient

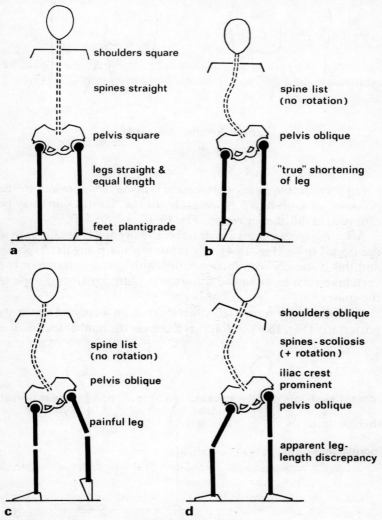

Fig. 18.2 (a) Normal posture, (b) short leg, (c) sciatic list, (d) scoliosis.

normal or "list": equal
prominence of erector spinae

scoliosis: rib hump or "bolster
sign" prominent

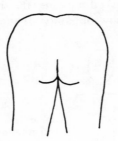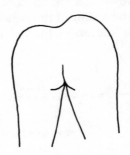

patient bending forwards

Fig. 18.3 'Bolster' sign.

bends forward the rotational element is made more obvious by the presence of a rib hump on one side, or the 'bolster sign' may be observed in the lumbar region (Fig. 18.3).

A *kyphosis* is an excessive dorsal convexity and is usually seen in the dorsal spine (Fig. 18.4). A *kyphus* is a sharp angular kyphosis and this is usually seen in association with collapse of one or two vertebrae such as occurs with fracture or inflammatory disease of the spine.

Lordosis is the term used when there is an increased concavity posteriorly (Fig. 18.4). A lordosis is seen in the lumbar region. It is

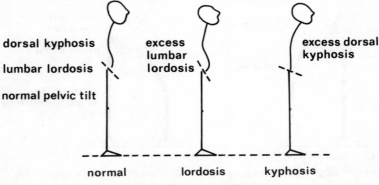

dorsal kyphosis

lumbar lordosis

normal pelvic tilt

excess
lumbar
lordosis

excess dorsal
kyphosis

normal   lordosis   kyphosis

Fig. 18.4 Kyphosis and lordosis.

commonly a postural defect but may be seen in a pronounced form with spondylolisthesis.

Pelvic obliquity indicates lateral tilting of the pelvis. It may result from a short leg or from a structural scoliosis.

Patients with pelvic obliquity who are in wheelchairs are liable to develop pressure sores over the more prominent buttock.

The *movements* tested are:

Forward flexion, which occurs in both the lumbar and dorsal spine. Many people are able to touch the floor with the tips of their fingers with the legs straight, but there is considerable variation in the normal range of movement. It should be noted if there is any pain or limitation of movement. Any rigidity of any area of the dorsal or lumbar spine should be detected. Patients with degenerative disease of the lumbar spine frequently have a very rigid spine and most of the forward flexion takes place at the hip joints (Fig. 18.5).

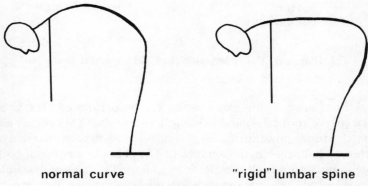

normal curve   "rigid" lumbar spine

Fig. 18.5   Forward flexion.

Extension movement is limited in various lesions, e.g. ankylosing spondylitis. Patients who have intersegmental instability will complain particularly on extension of the spine. The whole extension movement from the forward flexed position should be studied.

Lateral flexion. This is a sideways bend and the movement occurs mainly in the lumbar region.

Rotation. A rotation movement occurs in the dorsal spine, at the pelvis and the hip joints.

Examination with the patient lying supine

The straight leg raising test should be carried out with the foot plantar flexed and then dorsiflexed. This test puts the sciatic nerve on stretch and is positive if its component roots are involved. In most patients, the straight leg raising can be taken to 90° without discomfort (Fig. 18.6a).

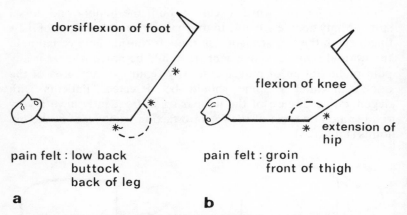

Fig. 18.6   (a) Straight leg raising test, (b) femoral stretch test.

A brief *neurological* examination can be performed. The knee jerk (nerve root L3-4) and ankle jerk (nerve root S1) reflexes are tested. Muscle power in the lower limb is tested, in particular that of extensor hallucis longus (nerve root L5). Muscle wasting of both thigh muscles and calf muscles is measured. The leg length should be measured. Sensory loss is determined, particularly light touch, over the dermatomes L4, L5, S1 (Fig. 18.7).

The hip joints should be examined. The abdomen can also be examined at this time.

Examination with the patient prone

The patient lies face downwards fully relaxed with a pillow under his pelvis.

Palpation of the whole spine should include individual spines and interspinous areas and the sacroiliac joints. Tender areas are noted (it must be remembered that there is a considerable overlap of nerve supply of the posterior primary rami and that tenderness at

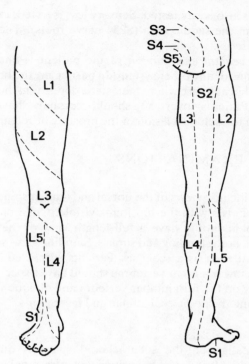

Fig. 18.7   Dermatomes of the lower limb.

any particular segment does not necessarily mean that there is any abnormality in that segment).

Deformities can be palpated, in particular, a kyphus or any excessive gap between spinous processes. In spondylolisthesis there may be a palpable step at the site of the forward slip.

The femoral stretch test consists of flexing the knee and then hyperextending the hip joint thus stretching the femoral nerve. It is positive if the patient complains of pain in the groin and thigh and indicates a possible high lumbar disc lesion (Fig. 18.6b).

Elderly patients will complain of back pain on performing this manoeuvre and this is not a positive response.

A brief *neurological* examination of the lower limb is performed. Muscle wasting of the glutei, hamstrings or calves is noted. Weakness of the gastrocnemius-soleus complex (S1-S2 nerve root) can be tested by plantar flexion of the foot. Weakness of the hamstrings is also easily tested. Sensory loss is tested, in particular, light touch in the saddle area (S234 nerve roots). The anal blink reflex is elicited.

Finally a *general examination* of the patient is undertaken to exclude lesions of any other system. In particular, the breast should be examined in any case where metastatic deposits in the spine are a possibility Patients over 50 should certainly have a rectal examination to exclude a lesion of the prostate or rectum.

SPECIAL EXAMINATIONS

Plain X-ray
This should include views of the dorsal and lumbar spine and an AP view of the pelvis with the hip joints visible. Children presenting with back pain should have a full length view of the dorsal and lumbar spine both standing and supine. Standing view will show any malalignment such as a scoliosis. Patients suspected of having a lesion of the lower lumbar vertebrae should have a specially centred lateral X-ray on the fifth lumbar vertebra and oblique views of this area to outline the pedicles, laminae and facet joints.

Myelogram
In this investigation the subarachnoid space is outlined with radiopaque dye. It is useful to exclude any intraspinal lesion higher than that suspected. It also may outline a disc protrusion. This examination does have its complications and should not be done as a routine measure. Its use should be restricted to those patients who are being considered for definite treatment. Lateral disc protrusions may not show on a myelogram as the lesion is too far lateral for the dye in the subarachnoid column to be indented.

Discogram
This investigation consists of injecting radiopaque material into the disc. The normal disc will only take up a small amount of the injected material but a degenerate disc will permit a larger injection. It may actually be demonstrated that the material can leak out of a disc. This investigation also has its share of complications. Unfortunately it demonstrates only that the disc is abnormal and this is a very frequent occurrence particularly in older patients. Such an abnormal disc may be symptomless and a discogram therefore has a high proportion of false positive results.

Intraspinal venogram
This investigation can also be used to outline the vertebral canal and its contents.

Blood test
A full blood count and sedimentation rate should be taken if there is any doubt that the patient may be suffering from a tumour, infection or ankylosing spondylitis. If the sedimentation rate is normal it is unlikely to be any of these. If there is any doubt, it should be repeated.

Various biochemical tests are useful in certain cases. An acid phosphatase should be taken if a carcinoma of the prostate is suspected. Serum calcium, serum phosphate and alkaline phosphatase should be performed if the patient exhibits any osteoporosis, as it may prove to be osteomalacia. Patients with myeloma may present with back pain and a battery of tests can be performed to exclude it.

Bone scan
A plain X-ray of the lumbar spine may show no abnormality in patients with tumours or infections for a considerable period of time. A more sensitive index of such abnormalities is the bone scan. Radioactive material is taken up more quickly in vascular regions affected by tumour or infection. These will appear as an area of increased radioactivity.

A bone scan is a useful screening test for metastases in bone.

DIFFERENTIAL DIAGNOSIS OF BACK PAIN

A patient whose primary complaint is back pain will have some lesion in the back; patients with back pain due to lesions elsewhere will have additional relevant signs and symptoms.

Non-spinal causes
Cardiovascular – myocardial infarct, dissecting aneurysm.
Respiratory – pleurisy, etc.
Gastrointestinal – carcinoma of the pancreas, penetrating gastric ulcer, carcinoma of the rectum.
Urological – kidney disease, carcinoma of the bladder.
Gynaecological – dysmenorrhoea, carcinoma of the body of the uterus.

Spinal causes
These can be classified as follows:

Tumour.
Infection.
Inflammatory.
Metabolic.
Discogenic.
Degenerative.
Traumatic.
Structural.
Mechanical.
Coccydinia.

Tumours
Tumours of the vertebral column may occur in the vertebrae or in the spinal canal (extradural or intradural tumours).

The commonest tumour is a *secondary deposit* in a vertebra (see Fig. 18.6, p. 154). Patients may present with acute back pain from a pathological fracture or with persistent back pain which keeps them awake at night. Secondary deposits tend to occur in the body of the vertebra and may erode the pedicles. When the body of the vertebra has been sufficiently weakened, a pathological fracture may result. The X-ray signs in vertebrae occur late and bone scan should be done if a secondary deposit is suspected in the vertebral column. Patients will usually have a raised sedimentation rate. When diagnosed the treatment consists of bed rest for acute pain. A local lesion should be treated with radiotherapy and if there are more general lesions chemotherapy should be prescribed.

Myelomatosis may present initially as a vertebral lesion in a manner similar to secondary metastases, as a pathological fracture or with persistent back pain. It is a generalised condition and a skeletal survey will reveal other lesions. There are typical abnormalities to be found on full blood examination and biochemistry. A bone marrow examination will confirm the diagnosis.

Osteoporosis of the spine will have a very similar presentation; the diagnosis of this condition depends to a large extent on the exclusion of other possibilities.

Primary bone tumours occur in the spine but infrequently. It is one of the more common sites for an osteoblastoma. These patients will complain of a persistent back pain even at rest and at a later stage will suffer the signs and symptoms of cord and nerve root compression.

TUMOURS OF THE SPINAL CANAL
These are usually extradural and the commonest lesion is a secondary metastasis.

Intradural tumours may be benign such as a meningioma or neurofibroma. Various types of gliomata are described as occurring within the spinal cord and are usually seen in young people.

Patients with tumours in the spinal canal have a variable presentation. They may have very severe back pain causing such distress that the patient may appear to be irrational and in danger of being considered 'functional'. Some have very little pain and present with neurological symptoms of weakness, numbness, or enuresis. They may present with deformities such as pes cavus or scoliosis.

The treatment of these lesions is usually surgical, excision of the tumour if possible, decompression of the spinal canal if it is not.

Infections of the vertebral column
Staphylococcal infection can occur producing an osteomyelitis of the vertebral body. The commonest area affected is adjacent to the disc. Patients complain of quite severe back pain and are pyrexial. The pain occurs at night and often keeps the patient awake. Such patients will have a raised white count and sedimentation rate; they may well have a positive blood culture.

X-ray will show the lesion adjacent to the disc space. As it progresses, the bodies become progressively eroded and will collapse anteriorly. An angular deformity or kyphosis results.

Unfortunately the staphylococcus is often only attenuated by inadequate antibiotic treatment. Infections of the spine may present therefore as a rather low grade persistent back pain. Patients have a raised sedimentation rate and X-ray changes again appear late, some two or three months after the onset of the condition.

Tuberculosis occurs in the spine. It is rarely seen in patients from western countries. However, it is frequently seen in under-developed countries. The lesion is at a similar site to staphylococcal infection. It may be accompanied by a considerable bone destruction and abscess formation (see Fig. 6.2, p. 23).

The spinal cord can be damaged by the abscess, by the

development of a kyphus and by loss of blood supply to the cord. Tuberculosis is sometimes accompanied by the formation of a large abscess. This may accumulate around the kidney as a perinephric abscess or along the psoas muscle and present in the groin as a psoas abscess.

TREATMENT
The usual treatment is an antibiotic to cure the infection. It is traditional to immobilise the patient in bed until the disease is quiescent. If there is persistent infection after a reasonable period of time, it is assumed that there is a sequestrum (an area of infected dead bone) in the vertebral column and operative exploration accompanied by spinal fusion is undertaken.

Ankylosing spondylitis
Ankylosing spondylitis is an inflammatory condition of the vertebral column. It occurs in young men who present with persistent back pain and a very stiff spine. On examination there is a rigid vertebral column, in particular extension movement is lost. Chest expansion is also decreased.

X-ray initially will show the sacro-iliac joints with a fluffy outline. As the disease progresses, ankylosis occurs firstly in the anterior longitudinal ligament and then the facet joints and the interspinous ligaments. Eventually these ligaments appear ossified giving the appearance of a bamboo spine.

The condition is of an uncertain prognosis. Some patients appear to have only a sacro-iliitis. Other patients become crippled with a rigid spine which unfortunately may be flexed. In some even the hip joints and the shoulder joints may be affected by the disease.

It is found that immobilisation tends to make these patients excessively stiff. Worse still, they tend to stiffen in the flexed position – so that when standing and walking, the head faces the ground. Ideally they should be kept active. The anti-inflammatory drug phenylbutazone reduces their symptoms and makes this possible. When the patient sleeps at night, he should be advised to lie flat on a firm bed with no pillow.

Some patients with advanced flexion deformities have undergone a spinal osteotomy to correct this.

Metabolic diseases
The condition of *osteoporosis* frequently presents in the spine.

These patients are commonly elderly ladies who have a decreased bone mass; however, the osteoid present is fully mineralised. They complain of chronic persistent backache and every so often may have a sudden severe episode of back pain associated with a crushed fracture of a vertebra. As time passes, they have a gradually increasing kyphosis and a decrease in overall height. They also have an increased tendency to fractures at other sites.

The condition of osteoporosis is characterised by a general decrease in bone substance but there is no biochemical defect or abnormality to be detected. X-ray will show rarified vertebrae. It may also show crush fractures. Sometimes the discs appear to be expanded into the vertebrae, the so-called 'fish-tail spine' (see Fig. 5.2, p. 16).

Patients with osteomalacia have a similar appearance in their spine and this should be excluded by biochemical tests. Osteomalacia of course is treatable. Patients with myelomatosis have a very similar appearance to those with osteoporosis. This should also be excluded by investigations. Patients on steroid therapy and patients with Cushing's disease develop osteoporosis and may have similar back symptoms.

TREATMENT
There is no specific treatment for this condition. Anabolic steroids and calcium fluoride have been prescribed and may afford relief. It is important to keep the patient active and if possible increase this activity. Supplements of vitamin D and calcium are usually prescribed.

Patients with acute pain from a recently collapsed vertebra may require bed rest for a few days. Those with chronic back pain are sometimes helped by a lumbosacral corset.

INTERVERTEBRAL DISC LESIONS
(see Fig. 12.3, p. 70)

An intervertebral disc is interposed between the bodies of adjacent vertebrae. In the young it consists of a central gelatinous nucleus pulposus surrounded by a strong annulus fibrosus. Separating it from the cancellous vertebral body is a layer of hyaline cartilage. It acts as a buffer between the vertebral bodies and permits a certain amount of movement to occur at each segment.

As the patient becomes older, 'degenerative changes' in the disc occur. At the molecular level there is:

1. Decrease in water content.

2. Alteration in type of glycosamino-glycan. There tends to be a decrease in chondroitin sulphate content and an increase in keratin sulphate.

3. Probably an alteration in the type and degree of maturity of constituent collagen.

In general the disc tends to become of more uniform consistency altering from a 'sealed fluid bearing' to one of generalised rubbery consistency.

As these changes occur, the disc is liable to damage from quite minor trauma. A compression force may cause a rupture of the hyaline cartilage and permit nucleus material to enter the cancellous bone of a vertebral body. This appears on X-ray as a spherical radiolucency – a Schmorl's node. It is one of the earlier indications of degenerative disc disease.

Such a disc will be less efficient mechanically and the whole segment of the spine will be weakened.

If the fibrous tissue of the annulus is degenerative, it is liable to crack. Minor trauma, especially of a twisting nature, will permit nucleus material to protrude through the cracks of the degenerative annulus. If this protrusion occurs posteriorly, the nucleus material is liable to progress lateral to the posterior ligament and impinge on nerve roots causing sciatic pain.

Intervertebral disc degeneration can be responsible for certain signs and symptoms:

1. Low back pain:

From the formation of Schmorl's nodes.

From pressure on the posterior longitudinal ligament.

From deranged segmental mechanisms due to disc dysfunction and eventually narrowing. This will produce some degree of subluxation at the facet joint and result in instability of the segment.

2. Nerve root pain. If disc material impinges on a nerve root, it may cause severe pain in the distribution of that nerve root (sciatica if the nerve root is L5 or S1). Initially the nerve root is inflamed and swollen; if the lesion persists, perineural fibrosis occurs.

3. Nerve root signs. These occur when the nerve root is compressed and loss of function due to damage of the nerve root can be demonstrated. Such nerve root compression can occur:

From a large disc protrusion compressing the nerve root in the spinal canal.

From a sequestrated portion of a disc protrusion compressing a nerve root in the intervertebral foramen.

From perineural fibrosis as can occur from a neglected or recurring disc protrusion. It can also occur after surgery.

From a massive disc prolapse which may compress the cauda equina. (These patients may present with bladder symptoms (retention of urine) as well as other signs.)

Patients with significant nerve root signs may require exploration of the lesion by operation.

Treatment

Unfortunately treatment affords only partial relief of symptoms. The following may be tried:

1. Rest. Complete rest in bed with adequate pain relief will rapidly relieve acute symptoms. It is also effective for acute recurrences. Partial rest by splintage with a plaster jacket or corset is of value.

2. Epidural injections. These are most effective in the early stages of nerve root pain. Local anaesthetic and steroid is instilled in the epidural space around the inflamed nerve root. This combined with some degree of immobilisation can afford quite dramatic and prolonged relief of symptoms.

3. Patients with chronic disc disease should be advised to avoid factors which precipitate symptoms, such as stooping and twisting movements of the back and repeated heavy lifting. Unfortunately many unskilled labouring jobs demand just such movements. Patients with disc disease cannot manage such work at the pace demanded of them by their employers.

4. A variety of non-specific treatments are found to be of value in some patients with intervertebral disc lesions.

5. Surgery may be indicated for persistent pain unrelieved by conservative measures. It may be indicated if there are significant nerve root signs. Emergency surgery is mandatory to relieve cauda equina compression (retention of urine).

LUMBAR NERVE ROOT LESIONS

These can be caused by:

1. Intervertebral disc protrusion (Fig. 18.8). The discs most

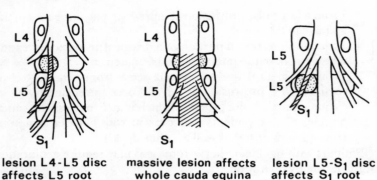

| lesion L4-L5 disc affects L5 root | massive lesion affects whole cauda equina | lesion L5-S$_1$ disc affects S$_1$ root |

Fig. 18.8   Lumbar disc lesions.

usually involved are L4-5 and L5-S1 but higher discs may also cause significant protrusions. The nerve root affected is usually one level distal to the protrusion. An L5 nerve root lesion is most frequently produced by an L4-5 disc. A sequestrated portion of disc may involve a root in the intervertebral foramen. A massive disc protrusion will affect all the nerve root at its level, including S234 nerve roots which supply the detrusor muscle of the bladder.

2.   Advanced degenerative changes in the spine. Osteophytes are formed from advanced degenerative changes of the disc or the facet joints. These are liable to compress the nerve root as it passes in the intervertebral foramen (Fig. 18.9).

3.   Spondylolisthesis (Fig. 18.10). In this condition a segment is so unstable that it is possible for the vertebra above to slip forward on the one below. These patients usually have low back pain, but

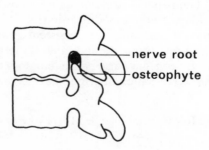

Fig. 18.9   Osteophyte causing nerve root canal stenosis.

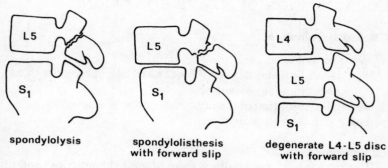

Fig. 18.10 Spondylolisthesis.

often have nerve root pain and sometimes transient nerve root signs.

4. Vertebral canal stenosis (Fig. 18.11). These patients have a narrowed vertebral canal due to:

Morphology – the canal may be of unusual shape.

Developmental factors such as achondroplasia.

Paget's disease.

Usually degenerative changes with in-growth of osteophytes into the canal.

Iatrogenic factors secondary to spinal fusion.

Patients complain of severe but vague back pain referred usually to both legs. This is often worse on exercise (spinal claudication). The nerve roots may be sufficieny compressed in the spinal canal to produce a cauda equina lesion.

5. Spinal tumours or infections.

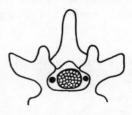
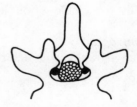

Fig. 18.11 Vertebral stenosis.

LOCALISATION OF NERVE ROOT SIGNS

Clinical examination

S1 nerve roots lesions
  Weakness of plantar flexion of foot and of lateral hamstrings.
  Weakness of gluteus maximus.
  Decreased sensation of the outer side and sole of foot.
  Ankle jerk depressed or absent.

L5 nerve root
  Weakness of extensor hallucis (also of medial hamstrings and of toe extensors).
  Wasting of calf muscles.
  Decreased sensation of outer side of calf and dorsum of foot.

L4 nerve root
  Weakness of tibialis anterior.
  Decreased sensation on inner side of lower leg.
  Decreased knee jerk.

S234 nerve roots
  Bladder dysfunction and lax anus.
  Saddle anaesthesia.
  No anal blink reflex.

Investigations

Myelogram
The subarachnoid space is outlined with radiopaque medium. A disc prolapse is seen as an indentation on the myodil column. It is a useful test to exclude serious lesions such as intraspinal tumours.

Electromyography
Electromyography will determine more accurately the muscles affected.

SEGMENTAL INSTABILITY

Certain patients have either persistent back pain on activity or recurrent bouts of severe back pain.

Many of these patients have a demonstrable cause for instability such as a disc lesion or spondylolisthesis.

Spondylolisthesis (Fig. 18.10)
Spondylolisthesis is a condition which permits a lumbar vertebra to slip forward on the one below. It is such a common condition that its significance is disputed. Many people with spondylolisthesis complain of no back symptoms at all. Various types are described:

1. Pars interarticularis defect
These patients may present with back pain in adolescence or early adult life. X-ray reveals a defect in the lamina between the superior and inferior facets of the vertebra. An oblique X-ray is frequently necessary to demonstrate the lesion.

A spondylolysis is the term used for a demonstrable pars interarticularis defect with no slip.

It is possible that the defect represents a stress fracture. Cases have occurred where the lesion has healed spontaneously.

Treatment should be conservative for as long as possible. Acute pain can be relieved by bed rest or a plaster jacket. Activities are monitored to avoid precipitating factors. Back exercises are of value to build up protecting muscles. A spinal fusion should only be done if the symptoms are intolerable, and the lesion is found to be confined to the area concerned.

2. Degenerative spondylolisthesis
A slip of a vertebra on the one below can occur in association with degenerative changes in the intervening disc and facet joints. This lesion is usually seen in middle age and the slip is usually of L4 on L5. The treatment is essentially conservative and a back brace is often very effective.

3. Congenital spondylolisthesis
This is associated with a defect of the posterior elements of the spine. This is not common, and presents in children as a marked lordosis.

4. Traumatic spondylolisthesis

5. Spondylolisthesis associated with fragilitas ossium

MANAGEMENT OF BACK PAIN

There are two main types of back lesions, those which can be diagnosed and those which cannot. Those which cannot be diagnosed demand sympathetic treatment which is empirical and therefore unsatisfactory. Even those patients who do demonstrate a significant lesion cannot always be relieved of their symptoms. In some cases this 'lesion' is so common as to be almost a normal occurrence. Therefore the presence of any particular lesion cannot lightly be assumed to be the whole cause of the patient's symptoms.

All patients who present with back pain are functional to some degree. In many this functional overlay is minimal. However, in many it adds considerably to the complaint. Even patients who have a demonstrable lesion to account for their symptoms are very difficult to assess and treat.

All patients presenting with back pain require careful history taking and full clinical examination. The management of such patients can be considered in various categories:

1. Mild symptoms only
Analgesic and anti-inflammatory drugs such as acetylsalicylic acid.

2. Acute symptoms
Patient cannot work or manage usual duties.
    Bed rest to relieve acute symptoms with pain relieving drugs (splintage with plaster jacket etc. if bed rest not possible).
    Mobilisation, with trunk, abdominal and back exercises.
    Placebo physiotherapy.
    Plain X-ray.
    Return to work.

3. Persistent and recurring back pain
These patients require full examination with X-ray, blood count, etc.
    If undiagnosable, treat sympathetically.
    If diagnosable treat conservatively:
        Analgesic and anti-inflammatory drugs (acetylsalicylic acid, indomethacin).
        Advice as regards activities.
        Physiotherapy
            Placebo treatment.

Back, trunk and abdominal exercises.
Advice on lifting and other activities.

4. Back pain and sciatica
For acute symptoms, treat as for acute back pain. If symptoms persist, bed rest and traction in hospital may be necessary. Further conservative management may include splintage with a plaster jacket.

Persistent symptoms require investigation with myelogram X-ray to define the lesion and exclude an associated lesion.

Epidural infiltration at the site of the lesion with local anaesthetic and steroid followed by immobilisation may afford worthwhile relief of symptoms.

Most patients will resolve with conservative management. Surgery is indicated only if nerve root involvement can be identified and the patients have:

Persistent nerve root pain.

Marked nerve root signs or increasing nerve root signs.

Cauda equina lesions with retention of urine, as an emergency operation.

OPERATIONS ON THE LUMBAR SPINE

Laminectomy
Laminectomy means partial or complete removal of the lamina of the vertebra (Fig. 18.12a). The object is to relieve nerve root pressure (causing sciatica) due to a disc protrusion. It will not relieve back pain due to instability, and may well make it worse.

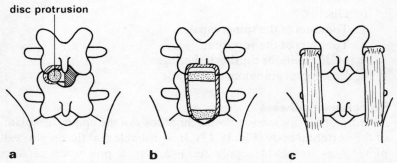

Fig. 18.12 Lumbar spine operations, (a) fenestration laminectomy, (b) decompression laminectomy, (c) intertransverse fusion.

Decompression

Decompression involves complete removal of the lamina of several vertebrae and exposing the cauda equina and nerve roots (Fig. 18.12b). The object is to decompress the nerve roots. It is of value when treating vertebral stenosis or tumours or infections.

Spinal fusion

The object of spinal fusion is to stabilise an unstable segment or segments of the spine (Fig. 18.12c). It is technically difficult and there is a high failure rate of obtaining a sound fusion of more than two segments. Spinal fusions are usually confined to the lower two spaces. Before embarking on a fusion operation, it is necessary to demonstrate the site of instability. It is also necessary to demonstrate that there is no disc disease proximally as this may well be made symptomatic by the extra strain of the adjacent fusion mass.

BACK CONDITIONS IN CHILDREN

Children, unlike adults, rarely complain of their backs. Therefore if they do, the complaint should be taken seriously and the child properly examined and fully investigated.

Children suffer from a great many lesions of their backs. These can be listed in order of prevalence as follows:
1. Scheurmann's disease.
2. Scoliosis.
3. Spondylolisthesis.
4. Prolapsed intervertebral disc.
5. Infections.
6. Discitis.
7. Tumours of the spinal canal.
8. Tumours of the vertebrae.
9. Malformations causing tethering.
10. Eosinophil granuloma.

Scheurmann's disease

Scheurmann's disease is an osteochondrosis of the epiphyseal plate of the vertebral body (Fig. 18.13). It is probable that the epiphyseal plate loses its blood supply secondary to a protrusion of disc material through the cartilage plate. The epiphyseal plate tends to fragment and growth of the front part of the vertebral body is

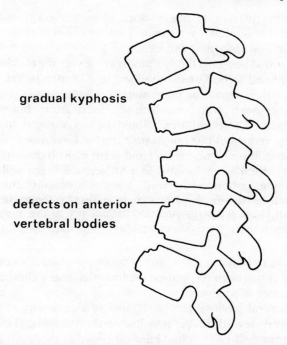

gradual kyphosis

defects on anterior
vertebral bodies

Fig. 18.13   Osteochondrosis of spine (Scheurmann's disease).

affected so that a gradual kyphosis occurs. The disc itself becomes
narrow and in the later stages is obviously degenerate.

These patients usually present in adolescence and this condition
is also known as adolescent kyphosis. They complain of either
dorsal or lumbar back pain. On examination there is a considerable
amount of spasm of the muscles of the spine and all movements are
limited. The straight leg raising also may be limited on each side.
There are no neurological signs. In the later stages the patients will
gradually develop an obvious kyphosis. X-rays will show the
irregularity of the epiphyseal plates in the dorsal spine. If the
disease is in the lumbar spine, the condition is manifested as an
irregularity in the anterior part of the vertebra. In the later stages
the vertebrae appear to be wedge shaped and the disc space
narrowed.

The causes of the condition are unknown. Some of the patients
are very athletic children who indulge in competitive sports, some

of them perform quite heavy work at an early age and it may therefore be related to trauma. However some cases occur in particularly lackadaisical children.

In the initial stages, if the symptoms are severe the child may need to be confined to bed or immobilised in a plaster jacket. Even in mild cases they should be prevented from indulging in competitive and contact sports. Not so much on account of injury, but to prevent over-fatigue. These children should be encouraged to take up swimming and should be taught postural back exercises.

If the condition is more severe and there is an obvious round back deformity, then a few months in a Milwaukee brace will show an improvement, often quite rapid. Very occasionally, the patients have such a severe kyphosis that operative correction using Harrington rods is necessary.

Scoliosis
A structural scoliosis is a quite common disease occurring in children. It has been recognised recently that many children have a minor degree of scoliosis.

A structural scoliosis can be defined as a deformity of the spine with lateral deviation and rotation of the vertebra. This can be demonstrated when the child bends forward as there is either a rib hump or bolstering on the convex side in the lumbar region (see Fig. 18.3). Furthermore the curve will still be present. When patients who have a so-called postural scoliosis or list bend forwards, the scoliosis is eradicated and there is no bolstering or rib hump.

These patients present because their parents notice the back deformity. Sometimes the parents notice that one buttock is more prominent than the other and this is observed particularly when the child appears in jeans or in a bathing suit. It is rare for the child to complain of any symptoms. If he does complain of back pain then a careful search should be instituted for any neurological signs.

A child with scoliosis should have a neurological examination of his lower limbs as well as of his back. The leg lengths should be measured and there should be a full length standing X-ray of the dorsal and lumbar spines. In the early stages, lateral X-rays are also necessary.

Causes
1. Congenital.
2. Infantile.

Benign.
Progressive.
3. Idiopathic, juvenile.
4. Neurological due to muscle imbalance; poliomyelitis, meningomyelocele, cerebral palsy.
5. Miscellaneous; neurofibromatosis, mid brain lesions, spinal tumour, etc.

Management
Mild cases of scoliosis should be kept under careful observation and should have a full length standing X-ray, certainly every two years, and every year when growth is rapid. Most of the types of scoliosis, except for some of the infantile cases, are progressive and the progression occurs most rapidly during the growth spurt.

If the curve is progressing significantly, then this is an indication for bracing the child. This progression usually occurs just before or after puberty (10–14). The brace used is the Milwaukee brace which fits snugly on the iliac crests and also has pressure applied to the occiput through a pad (Fig. 18.14). In front there is a throat piece which keeps the head extended and held against the occipital pad. The brace extends from the occiput to the iliac crest. If there is a rib hump then pressure can be applied to that via the pads. Properly applied a Milwaukee brace is a very efficient method of controlling scoliosis and some devotees claim that it can partially correct a curve.

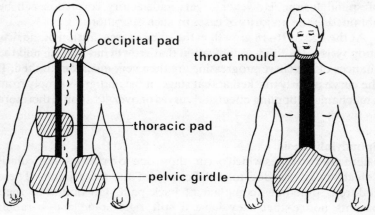

Fig. 18.14 Milwaukee brace.

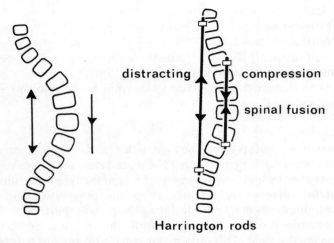

distracting   compression

spinal fusion

Harrington rods

Fig. 18.15   Harrington rods in operative treatment of scoliosis.

Severe curves over 40° require to be stabilised, and if possible corrected. Stabilisation is by a very extensive spinal fusion which covers the whole length of the curve and beyond it. The correction can be obtained by various methods. One method involves the use of a Harrington rod which will jack the curve apart on the concave side; a further rod on the convex side can assist in the reverse direction (Fig. 18.15). This is an extensive operation and it does mean that the spine is rigid and growth of course ceases in the areas of spinal fusion. However a very satisfactory correction can be obtained in the majority of cases by such operations.

At the age of 16–18 growth in the spine ceases. Fusion of the iliac apophysis is taken as an indication that growth has ceased, and the chances of the curve progressing are then very much diminished. If the curve is fairly marked at that stage, it may progress simply from a mechanical toppling effect and curves of over 40° should therefore be fused.

Spondylolisthesis
There are two types which occur, those due to a pars interarticularis defect and those due to a deficiency of the facet joints. These children sometimes complain of back pain. On occasions their parents notice that they have a stiff rigid spine and a rather prominent lordosis and the buttocks are obvious. X-ray may show

quite severe slip, usually of the 5th lumbar vertebra on the sacrum. Cases with neurological complications have been described.

If the slip is not too severe and the patient does not have severe symptoms, it is usually sufficient to restrict his activities and prevent him from participating in competitive and contact sports. If there is pain a brace may help to relieve it. If the lesion is progressing, as shown by serial X-rays, and he is having a significant back pain, then a spinal fusion is indicated.

Prolapsed intervertebral discs
These occur less frequently in children than in adults. Again the patients do not complain particularly of their back. They may complain of sciatica and sometimes their mothers notice that they are standing with an obvious list and have a rigid spine. They may have neurological signs of the lower limbs.

These patients should be managed conservatively if possible and it may well be necessary for them to be admitted to hospital for bed rest and traction. They may require a considerable period of time in a plaster jacket before the symptoms resolve. Unfortunately quite often these lesions do not resolve and a laminectomy to relieve the symptoms may be necesssary.

Infective lesions of the spine
The most common site of an infective lesion is in the metaphyseal region of the vertebral body, i.e. adjacent to the epiphyseal cartilage plate. Quite often the disc is affected as well. The commoner infections are staphylococcal infections and tuberculosis. The treatment of these lesions is the same as for adults.

Discitis
This condition occurs in children probably more frequently than is recognised. The child has acute back pain with a rigid spine, and straight leg raising is often limited. He may be pyrexial and may have a raised white count and ESR. The lesion may be due to some subclinical infection but usually no organism can be identified. Initially X-ray will show no abnormality but at a later stage calcification may be noted in the disc and after two or three months there is obvious narrowing of the disc space and sclerosis of the surrounding bodies.

The symptoms usually subside rapidly with bed rest and

immobilisation in a plaster jacket. The differential diagnosis is an osteomyelitis of the vertebral body and, as this may be very difficult in the early stages, it is reasonable to treat these children with antibiotics as though they had a staphylococcal infection.

In the later stages, the disc space is obviously narrowed; apart from this, the child suffers no serious disability.

Intraspinal tumours
It must be remembered that these occur in children; unfortunately they are frequently mis-diagnosed in the early stages.

The commonest presenting symptoms are:
1. Back pain.
2. Enuresis.
3. Weakness of the lower limbs and limp.
4. Torticollis, scoliosis or kyphosis.

The physical signs may be difficult to detect initially. There may be limitation of back movements with spasm and rigidity but specific signs include:
1. Abnormal reflexes.
2. Spastic or flaccid paresis.
3. Sensory loss.
4. Scoliosis.

The types of lesion also are different from intraspinal tumours in adults. In adults the most common intraspinal tumours are neurofibroma and meningioma. In children the most common lesions appear to be intramedullary gliomata and other common lesions include neuroblastoma, secondary metastases and teratoma.

The investigations should include an X-ray; a plain X-ray may well show widening of the spinal canal. However the lesion is frequently more proximal than expected and a full length view of the dorsal and lumbar spine should be taken to exclude this. It is a wise precaution in investigating children with back lesions that a full length view of both dorsal and lumbar spines should be available. A myelogram of course is essential to localise a lesion. The CSF protein is raised in children with spinal tumours.

Treatment is by surgical operation, if possible to remove the lesion, or at least to decompress it. Laminectomy may have to be very extensive and sometimes stabilisation by spinal fusion is required if it is considered that the prognosis is good enough to warrant it.

Tumours of the vertebra

Tumours of the bones of the vertebra also occur and include lesions such as osteoblastoma and aneurysmal bone cysts.

Malformations causing tethering

When the child is born the spinal cord usually reaches the level of the third lumbar vertebra. In adults it reaches the level of the twelfth thoracic or first lumbar. There are certain lesions which tend to tether the spinal cord, such as spina bifida occulta, diffuse lipomata and diastematomyelia.

These children frequently present with foot deformities, the most common of which is pes cavus. In addition they have bladder problems, in particular enuresis. Both these ailments can be ascribed to traction on the terminal sacral roots, the S2, 3, 4. If the lesion is not diagnosed early, more severe paresis and irreversible damage to nerve function can occur. These lesions should be suspected in children with foot deformities, enuresis, and absent ankle reflexes and should be investigated with myelography. Surgical relief of these lesions can relieve the tethering and allow the child to develop normally.

Eosinophil granuloma

This is a condition which usually occurs in the dorsal or cervical vertebra. The child presents with pain in this region and X-ray shows gross wedging of the vertebra concerned. At one time this lesion was known as Calvé's disease because it was thought to be an osteochondrosis. It appears to be a benign lesion and the symptoms usually resolve satisfactorily.

CHAPTER 19

Hip Conditions

HISTORY TAKING

In adults the main symptoms relating to the hip are pain, stiffness and a limp.

Pain

Pain is the most important symptom. In taking the history certain facts must be elucidated:

The typical *site* for hip pain is usually the groin. It may also be felt in the thigh or the shin. The pain may radiate to these areas and to the greater trochanter and the buttock. Hip pain is frequently felt in the knee; this may be particularly confusing when treating children.

The site of the pain is important for differentiating from back pain which may often be felt in the buttock and the region of the greater trochanter with radiation down the back of the leg. Patients often use the word 'hip' as an euphemism for the buttock.

The *radiation* of pain must be determined. Hip pain may radiate from the groin down the thigh to the knee and even to the shin. It may also radiate to the greater trochanter and sometimes the buttock.

Pain with such radiation must be differentiated from pain from an upper lumbar disc, which may radiate down the front of the thigh towards the knee.

The pain may be *persistent* or *episodic*. It must be noted whether it occurs at rest or on activity. Pain in the hip joint from osteoarthritis is usually relieved by rest and worse on walking.

The *severity* of the pain must be assessed. Patients with pain keeping them awake at night demand active treatment. Such pain requires efficient investigation to exclude any lesion such as an infection or tumour. It is possible to determine the severity of pain by inquiring about the patient's use of analgesics and the effects of various forms of treatment.

Relieving factors must be determined such as analgesics, rest, activity. Exacerbating factors must be determined.

Stiffness or limitation of movement is another symptom of which patients may complain. Enquiries should be made about difficulties with dressing, particularly shoes and stockings. Patients have difficulties with sitting, and getting into and out of cars. Patients with very severe hip disease can be considerably incapacitated by stiffness.

Limp is an important symptom. Adult patients usually complain of pain and stiffness before complaining of their limp. However in children, limp is often the presenting symptom and a child who limps must be thoroughly examined and investigated to exclude the various forms of hip disease.

Any previous history of injury or any history of past symptoms in the hips must be determined. This is particularly important when dealing with medicolegal cases.

Any past treatment or previous investigations must be elucidated. Any particular effects of past treatment should be noted.

In children the age of the patient is important and a history of the birth and development from infancy should be determined. A history of growth milestones must be obtained, particularly the date at which walking occurred. Limp is one of the most important symptoms in a child, and if a history of limp is obtained in a child, the patient should be fully investigated.

In addition, the age of onset is important for certain conditions occur more commonly at certain ages. Perthes' disease is more common between the ages of three and eight years, whereas slipping of the upper femoral epiphysis is more common in the ages ten to fifteen years.

A child who complains of knee pain must be examined and investigated to exclude hip disease. These investigations should include an X-ray of the hips.

EXAMINATION

Examination of the hip joint (Fig. 19.1) should be performed with the patient stripped to the underpants. It should be conducted both standing and with the patient lying on his back.

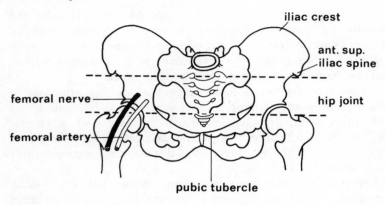

Fig. 19.1   Anterior view of the bony landmarks of the pelvis and hip joint.

Examination with the patient standing

Inspection of the spine and pelvic contours will detect any tilt of the pelvis. It is possible to see any obvious deformity or abnormal attitude of the lower limbs.

Gait. The patient should be observed walking and any abnormality of gait or limp detected.

Trendelenburg test is performed with the patient standing. This test depends on the efficiency of the abductors on the affected side. The patient stands on the good leg and as he does so, the pelvis on the opposite side is raised, thus demonstrating that the gluteus medius is working efficiently. He then stands on the affected leg and if there is inefficient action of the gluteus medius, the pelvis will sag on the opposite side (Fig. 19.2).

The causes of an abnormal Trendelenburg test are:

1. Weakness of the abductor muscles, as in polio or meningomyelocele.

2. Inefficiency of the fulcrum which permits the abductor muscles to work, as in congenital dislocation of the hip or subluxation of the hip.

3. A reflex inhibition of the abductor muscles due to pain in the hip joint on performing the test, as is found in some patients with osteoarthritis.

Examine the movements of the spine.

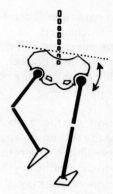

opposite side of pelvis raised by effective action of gluteus medius

a

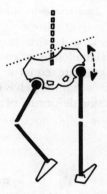

opposite side of pelvis sags because of ineffective action of gluteus medius

b

Fig. 19.2   Trendelenburg test, (a) negative, (b) positive.

Examination with the patient supine

Inspection

The patient is inspected for any deformities or abnormal attitudes of the lower limbs. Any obvious shortening is noted. The bony contours are noted, in particular the anterior superior iliac spines, iliac crests and greater trochanters.

The soft tissue contours are inspected for any obvious wasting or abnormal shape around the hip, buttocks and thighs.

Any scars or other abnormalities are noted.

Palpation

This includes palpation of the bony prominences. The most important of these are the two anterior superior iliac spines and by palpating these it is possible to align the pelvis and lower limbs. Palpation is also used to determine any points of tenderness around the hip joint. Skin temperature may also be determined. At this stage, the peripheral pulses should be palpated to exclude any vascular disease.

Measurement

The leg lengths are measured. The true leg length is measured from the anterior superior iliac spine to the medial malleolus on each side.

The apparent leg lengths are usually measured from the umbilicus to the medial malleolus on each side.

If the true leg lengths are equal and there is some apparent shortening, this indicates that the pelvis is tilted. The cause of this is probably due to adduction deformity of one of the lower limbs (Fig. 19.3).

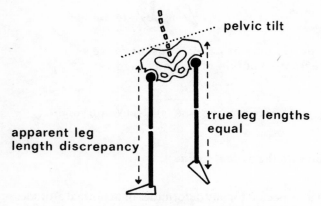

Fig. 19.3　Hip adduction deformity.

The girth of the quadriceps is measured on each side some twelve centimetres above the upper pole of the patella.

Movements of the hip joint
The active range of movement is determined first and then the passive range. The movements which occur at the hip joint are:
Flexion and extension (Fig. 19.4).
Abduction and adduction (Fig. 19.5).
Internal rotation and external rotation, which can be measured with the hip in extension and then in ninety degrees of flexion.

knee flexed

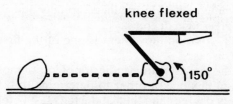

Fig. 19.4   Hip flexion range.

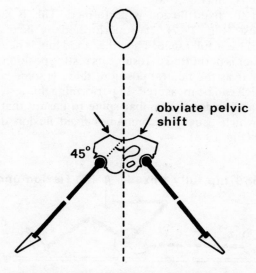

compare abduction both legs simultaneously
Fig. 19.5   Hip abduction range.

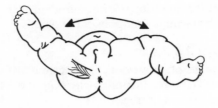

note spasm of adductors

Fig. 19.6   Hip abduction-in-flexion in children.

These movements are determined formally and the results can usually be expressed in degrees.

In the adult, rotation movement is one of the first to be lost in degenerative disease.

In a child, the most sensitive indicator of loss of movement is loss of abduction-in-flexion. In order to determine this, both hips are flexed to ninety degrees and then abducted. Just before the limit of abduction is reached in a painful hip, spasm will be observed in a child. Spasm is a reflex contraction of the adductors and occurs just before pain is felt (Fig. 19.6).

The test for fixed flexion is performed. This is known as the Thomas test (Fig. 19.7). It is performed by flexing both hips passively to their full range. Then the 'good hip' is held fully flexed and the other is permitted to resume its resting position. If it will not extend as far as the neutral position, there is some residual fixed flexion which can be measured. In performing this test, it is usual to put one hand under the lumbar spine to ensure that the lumbar lordosis (which usually accompanies fixed flexion deformity) is ironed out (Fig. 19.8).

"good" hip fully flexed   **hip flexion unmasked**

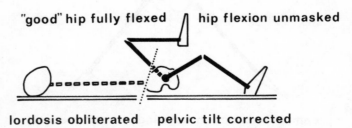

lordosis obliterated   pelvic tilt corrected

Fig. 19.7   The Thomas' test.

Finally, examine the knee joint, the abdomen and the pelvis to exclude any general cause of 'hip pain'.

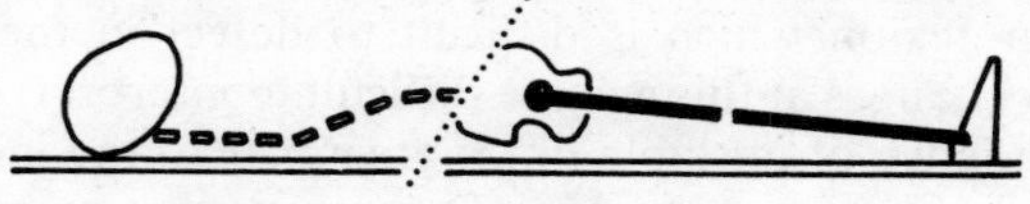

increased lordosis ⠂ hip flexion masked

increased pelvic tilt

Fig. 19.8   Hip flexion deformity.

CONGENITAL DISLOCATION OF THE HIP

This condition is found in children at birth or shortly afterwards. It is fairly common. The incidence of a definite dislocation of the hip is probably about three in two thousand births. The incidence of an 'unstable' hip at birth found by screening tests is higher.

Several factors are known about the incidence:

The incidence varies as to race (it is practically never found in Negroes).

It is found more commonly in Mediterranean countries than in northern Europe.

It is much more common in females than males (about 6:1).

It may be familial.

It is often associated with other deformities and abnormalities.

It is found frequently if the baby presents as a breech at birth.

The lesion is best diagnosed at birth and screening tests have been devised to make the diagnosis.

The Otolani test

This test consists of flexing the baby's hips to ninety degrees and then abducting them. The test is positive when abduction is accompanied by a definite palpable clunk as the head of the femur slips back into the acetabulum.

Demonstration of the unstable hip (Barlow)

This can be done by fixing the pelvis with one hand and with the other pressing the head and neck of femur backwards out of the acetabulum.

Combined test
It is best to demonstrate that the hip can be dislocated and then to reduce it using an Otolani test (Fig. 19.9).

It should be noted that if the hip is irreducible, then none of these tests will be positive. One has then to rely on limitation of abduction-in-flexion which is difficult to detect in the newborn child. X-ray changes at this age are difficult to interpret. It is found that the incidence of unstable hip is greater than the incidence of congenital dislocation of the hip. This means that many children born with unstable hips will stabilise themselves without resulting disability.

However it is possible to splint all children with unstable hips using simple apparatus. It has been shown conclusively that by doing so for about three months after birth, the incidence of congenital dislocation of the hip is much reduced and the treatment is very much simplified.

If the hip is allowed to remain dislocated, secondary changes will occur. The longer the hip remains dislocated, the more severe the

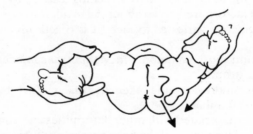

1. Steady "normal" limb
2. Adduct & push "abnormal" limb posteriorly

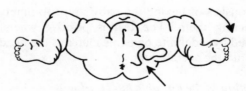

3. Abduct abnormal limb – hear & feel "clunk"

Fig. 19.9   Test for unstable hip at birth.

changes will be and the more difficult the lesion will be to treat. Bone abnormalities will occur:

Abnormalities of the femoral head, which may be misshapen; ossification will be delayed.

The acetabulum will become more shallow and more sloping; its alignment will be altered in relation to the head of the femur.

The femoral neck may be anteverted. The normal neck-shaft angle in the adult points just forward of the coronal plane. When the femoral neck is anteverted, the head and neck are pointing markedly forward in relation to the femoral shaft.

Abnormalities will occur in ligaments and muscles:

The adductor and psoas muscles will develop contractures inhibiting reduction.

The ligaments will be contracted possibly forming an hour-glass contracture between the head of the femur and the acetabulum.

A limbus can form (an inverted acetabular labrum).

Clinical diagnosis

The signs alter according to the age of the patient.

At birth the lesion is best diagnosed by a combination of the Otolani and Barlow tests as stated. There will be limitation of abduction with the hips flexed to ninety degrees.

Between six months and twelve months (Fig. 19.10) patients will have limitation of abduction-in-flexion; they may have a short leg; there may be an altered attitude of the lower limb (usually internal rotation).

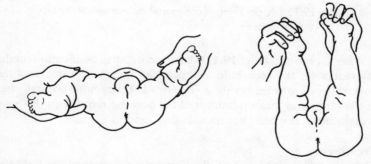

limitation of abduction in flexion   shortening of limb

Fig. 19.10   Test for congenital dislocation of the hip at a later age.

From twelve to eighteen months the diagnosis is easier and there are several indications. There may be delayed walking or even a significant limp (waddling gait). There may be a short leg. There will be limitation of abduction-in-flexion and altered skin creases.

In the older child the diagnosis is much easier, and all the physical signs outlined above will be more obvious. The child frequently presents with a significant limp which is a Trendelenburg limp with the pelvis sagging towards the affected side during weight bearing.

X-ray diagnosis
At birth special views have to be taken. This consists of abducting the legs to forty-five degrees and holding them in internal rotation. A line along the shaft of the femur will pass through the sacroiliac joint on the normal side and pass above it on the side with congenital dislocation of the hip.

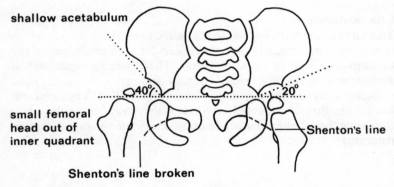

Fig. 19.11   X-ray signs of congenital dislocation of the hip.

After six months (Fig. 19.11) there is a delay in ossification on the affected side, the acetabulum slopes with increased angle, and the femoral neck may lie in valgus. The head of the femur normally lies in the inner and lower quadrant of the acetabulum. When the head is dislocated, the head lies outside this quadrant.

Treatment
This depends on the age at diagnosis; the younger the patient the more simple the treatment. However, after treatment the child must be kept under observation until maturity.

Diagnosed at birth

The hips should be held in the reduced position for at least three months by a splint. There are a variety of splints available. The most certain method is to fix the lower limbs in a plaster spica with the hips in rather more than ninety degrees of flexion and rather less than ninety degrees of abduction.

Other more aesthetically pleasing splints have the disadvantage of being less certain in holding the hips in the desired position. After three months the hips may be released but the child should be kept under observation and certainly have an X-ray at six months and at eighteen months. Observation should continue until maturity.

Diagnosis after six months of age means that the hip will have to be gradually reduced before treatment can start. This reduction is usually performed with skin traction. A gallows type of traction can be used and after a few days the hips are gradually abducted until the hip is reduced. Following this the legs are held in plaster and the plaster is maintained for about six months.

In the older child this method may fail to reduce the hips in which case an open operation will have to be done to place the head inside the acetabulum. At this age one or more of the various secondary pathological factors may be involved and have to be corrected (such as releasing the contracture of the hip ligaments or releasing tight adductors and psoas muscles). Two particular secondary pathological changes may require further operations.

Malalignment of the acetabulum can be corrected by an osteotomy through the pelvis just above the acetabulum (Fig. 19.12). A wedge of bone is placed into this osteotomy to alter the

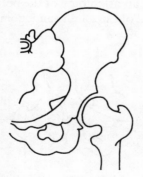
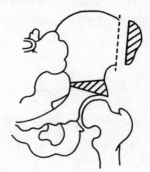

dysplasia of acetabulum   innominate osteotomy
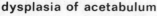
Fig. 19.12   Innominate osteotomy.

alignment of the acetabulum so that it better accommodates the head of the femur and the hip is made more stable. This operation is known as an innominate osteotomy.

Sometimes *anteversion of the neck of the femur* persists to such an extent that a rotational osteotomy of the upper shaft of the femur has to be performed. This permits the head and the neck to resume a stable position inside the hip joint with the rest of the lower limb in neutral rotation.

Early diagnosis and adequate treatment of congenital dislocation of the hip is essential. Failure of treatment means that these people have crippling symptoms in early adult life.

A patient with an unreduced dislocation of the hip will have a very ungainly limp and will develop osteoarthritis between the head of the femur and the side of the pelvis in the early thirties.

A patient with an inadequately treated dislocation of the hip will have a subluxing hip and will develop a painful osteoarthritis in the early twenties.

ACETABULAR DYSPLASIA

These patients may not have any of the signs of a dislocation of the hip. However, in adolescence they start developing symptoms of pain and a limp and X-ray will show that the acetabulum is 'shallow' and more sloping than normal (Fig. 19.13). If they are untreated, they almost certainly will develop osteoarthritis of the hip joint in their early twenties of such severity that they will require operative treatment.

These patients are best treated by an osteotomy of the pelvis to realign the acetabulum over the head of the femur (an innominate

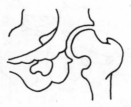
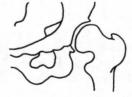

normal   dysplasia of acetabulum

Fig. 19.13   Acetabular dysplasia.

osteotomy). Another operation is to supplement the acetabulum by bone from the iliac crest. This again will afford a 'cover' for the head of the femur and prevent subluxation.

PERSISTENT FEMORAL NECK ANTEVERSION

These patients again will have none of the signs or symptoms of congenital dislocation of the hip but they are found to have anteversion of the femoral neck in relation to the femoral shafts (Fig. 19.14). As a result, in order for the head of the femur to be adequately contained in the acetabulum, the lower limbs have to be fully internally rotated.

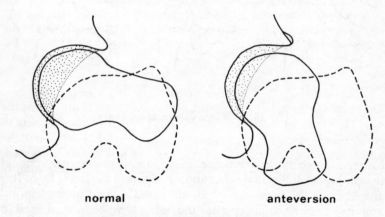

normal   anteversion

Fig. 19.14   Femoral neck anteversion.

These patients usually present with in-toeing. Persistent femoral neck anteversion is one of the common causes of an in-toe gait.

Usually this condition can be corrected by postural exercises and advice as to sitting. One of the main abnormalities with these children is sitting in the so-called television position, with hips and knees flexed and the lower limbs fully internally rotated. Children should be advised to sit with the hips externally rotated, i.e. in a cross-legged position. Rarely the condition is so severe and so persistent that a rotation osteotomy of the upper end of the femur is indicated. This allows the head of the femur to be well contained within the acetabulum with the limbs in neutral position.

COXA VARA

The normal angle between the neck and the shaft of the femur in the adult is about one hundred and thirty degrees. If this is significantly reduced, the condition known as coxa vara exists (Fig. 19.15). In some conditions, the angle is reduced to below ninety degrees and significant shortening of the lower limb results.

Congenital coxa vara is due to an abnormality of ossification of the neck of the femur. It is rare but can produce severe shortening. In order to correct the lesion, it is necessary to perform an osteotomy setting the lower limb in abduction relative to the neck.

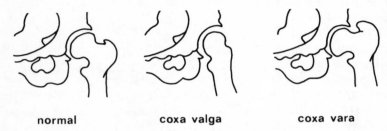

normal   coxa valga   coxa vara

Fig. 19.15   Coxa valga and coxa vara.

Congenital coxa vara is sometimes seen in association with proximal femoral focal defect and other abnormalities of the lower limb. It is also seen as the residuum of an untreated slipped upper femoral epiphysis, after trauma or after the bones have been weakened in growing children. Frequent causes nowadays are renal rickets and fibrous dysplasia.

PROXIMAL FEMORAL FOCAL DEFECT

These are an uncommon series of conditions which occur as congenital abnormalities in children. The upper end of the femur is affected to a varying degree. In addition to the lesion of the proximal end of the femur, in about 50 per cent of cases there is also an abnormality of the distal portion of the lower limb. The lesion may be bilateral or form part of a series of abnormalities of the other limbs.

These patients suffer varying degrees of absence or varying degrees of hypoplasia of the proximal portion of the femur. In the milder forms there may be just coxa vara and a rather short femur with the hip joint apparently normal. In the most severe forms there is no recognisable hip joint and the majority of the femur is absent.

As these children develop, they will have a very significant leg length discrepancy which can only be corrected by a prosthesis. Any surgical treatment required, therefore, is necessarily directed to fitting an efficient prosthesis.

TRAUMATIC SYNOVITIS OF THE HIP

This is a condition which occurs in children who present with a complaint of pain in the hip or knee and on examination are found to have limitation of hip movements.

The condition is usually found in boys and there may be a history of injury. The patient is noticed to have a limp and he may complain of pain in the hip or knee.

On examination there is limitation of movement in the affected hip and the most sensitive monitor of this limitation of movement is limitation of abduction of the hips flexed to ninety degrees.

All other investigations are negative. X-rays are normal, full blood count, and sedimentation rate show no abnormality. Patients with this condition have been subjected to a variety of investigations and no cause for the lesion has been discovered.

The condition resolves spontaneously. It is usual to keep the patient in bed for several days until hip movements return to normal. It is necessary to perform investigations to exclude lesions such as Perthes' disease and tuberculosis of the hip joint.

SEPTIC ARTHRITIS OF THE HIP

The pathology of this condition is much as described for septic arthritis of other joints. It is not common in the hip joint but it can cause crippling of the patient. The commonest causative organism is the staphylococcus but other bacteria may be involved. The disease may develop secondary to an osteomyelitis of the upper end of the femur. Direct spread from such a focus will involve the hip joint as the capsule is attached well distal to the epiphyseal plate (see Fig. 11.2, p. 60).

In the newborn and infants, septic arthritis of the hip may follow a generalised septicaemia. It may be noticed that the limb is no longer being moved. There may be some localised swelling or tenderness or obvious pain on movement in the affected hip. X-ray may show distension of the capsule as seen by examining the soft tissue shadows. The white blood count will be raised.

As the disease develops, the articular cartilage of the femoral head is extensively damaged, as may be the epiphysis and the growth plate. The pressure of fluid inside the joint will tend to extrude the head from the acetabulum. A secondary dislocation can therefore occur. The head may reform in due course and reossify but it will have an abnormal shape and abnormal function of the hip will almost certainly ensue.

In older children and adults, the disease is frequently associated with osteomyelitis of the neck of the femur. If the disease is unchecked the articular surface will be extensively damaged and adhesions will occur in the joint. Eventually a fibrous or a bony ankylosis will follow and the joint be wholly destroyed.

This condition demands early diagnosis and treatment. The diagnosis can be confirmed by aspiration of the hip under general anaesthetic – purulent fluid will be found. Treatment requires decompression of the hip joint. A window of capsule is removed to ensure adequate drainage. Relevant antibiotics are given and continued until the infection has resolved. The hip is splinted by traction in the early stages and later a plaster spica will be required to maintain the femoral head in position as healing is taking place. If treated early, the results can be excellent. If treated late, the results are disastrous.

PERTHES' DISEASE

Perthes' disease is an osteochondrosis – a degenerative (but reparable) condition of the epiphysis which is almost certainly due to repeated episodes of infarction (Fig. 19.16). These may be induced by trauma.

It occurs in the upper femoral epiphysis. It is most common in boys between the ages of three and eight years.

The patients present with limp and may complain of pain in the hip region or in the knee of the same side. On examination spasm is evident in the adductor muscles of the affected hip and there will be limitation of movement, particularly of abduction-in-flexion.

The diagnosis is made on X-ray. Other investigations are performed to exclude infective lesions which can mimic Perthes' disease.

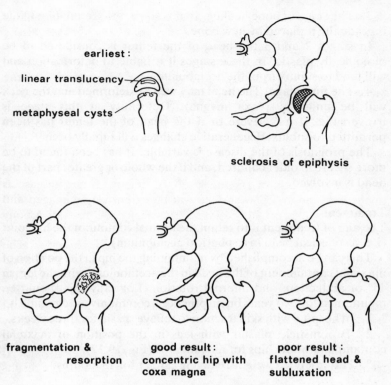

earliest:

linear translucency

metaphyseal cysts

sclerosis of epiphysis

fragmentation &
resorption

good result:
concentric hip with
coxa magna

poor result:
flattened head &
subluxation

Fig. 19.16   Changes in Perthes' disease.

The disease process lasts for over two years. If left untreated the head will become flattened and deformed and will tend to sublux from the acetabulum. Such a hip will rapidly develop symptomatic degenerative changes.

Various phases of the disease are described which can be monitored by serial X-rays:

1. The phase of necrosis of the femoral head. The affected bone dies. X-rays may show a linear translucency in the lateral film which is the earliest sign. Later the head will appear sclerotic and metaphyseal cysts will be seen along the growth plate.

2. The stage of revascularisation and resorption. The head appears to fragment and be reabsorbed on X-ray. The dead bone is replaced by granulation tissue.

3. The stage of bone healing. In this stage, the granulation tissue is gradually replaced by new bone.

In stages 2 and 3 the head of the femur is considered to be biologically plastic. In these stages it is liable to deformation and will tend to sublux from the acetabulum.

4. The final stage. The head may well be deformed and the neck will be enlarged (coxa magna). Deformity at this stage is irreversible. If it is severe or if the head of the femur has been permitted to sublux, degenerative changes will rapidly occur.

The prognosis of the disease is variable. It has been found to be more severe in older children, and if the whole or greater part of the head is involved.

Treatment

The aim of treatment is to retain the normal contour of the hip joint (i.e. a spherical head in a spherical acetabulum).

This can be accomplished by maintaining the hip in the position of maximal containment of the head in the acetabulum, with the legs in 45° of abduction, and internal rotation. Logically this should be maintained for two years but in practice a commonly used regime is:

1. In hospital with skin traction to relieve spasm for three weeks.

2. 'Broomstick' plaster with legs in the position of maximal containment of the hips for nine months (Fig. 19.17).

3. Patten-ended weight-relieving caliper for 15 months.

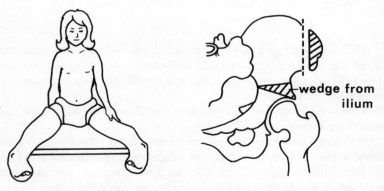

"broomstick" abduction plaster

innominate osteotomy

wedge from ilium

Fig. 19.17   Treatment of Perthes' disease.

Operative treatment may be undertaken to align the acetabulum so that the head of the femur is most efficiently contained. This is done by an innominate osteotomy.

In ideal conditions, this osteotomy is performed a few weeks after diagnosis. The child requires immobilisation afterwards for two or three months. He is then released and considered not to require further treatment. In successful cases, the convalscence is much reduced.

SLIPPED UPPER FEMORAL EPIPHYSIS

Slipped upper femoral epiphysis is a not uncommon condition in which the epiphysis slips posteriorly and downwards on the femoral neck. The separation occurs through the growth plate between the zones of hypertrophic and calcified cartilage. It is more common in boys than girls and the age range is 10–17 years (Fig. 19.18).

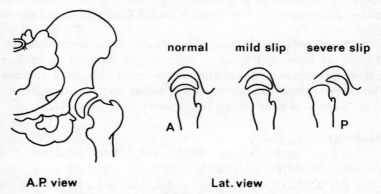

Fig. 19.18   Slipped upper femoral epiphysis.

The aetiology is uncertain. It occurs frequently in overweight boys so mechanical factors are important. It occurs occasionally in young athletes as an acute severe slip. Some patients have other growth plate deformities such as Madelung's deformity or genu recurvatum. It is seen in patients with scurvy, with rickets, and in cretinism.

X-ray is mandatory to diagnose and assess this condition. It is essential to have a good lateral view (axial) of the hip joint. The earliest sign is a slight slipping of the head of the femur on the neck. A slip of under one-third diameter in the lateral view is a mild slip. If it is more than one-third diameter it is a severe slip. AP X-rays are difficult to interpret in the early stages. A severe slip is more easily seen.

Clinically patients with slipped epiphysis will present:

1. As a mild subacute slip. These children will have a limp and complain of pain in the affected hip or the knee of the same side. On examination, they may show spasm in the adductor muscles of the affected hip. Other movements may be normal. A lateral hip X-ray will show a mild slip.

2. As a severe acute slip. These children will have severe pain after a moderate injury. They cannot walk. The leg lies in external rotation and adduction (like a fracture of the neck of the femur). They may have a previous history of a subacute slip. A lateral X-ray will demonstrate a severe slip.

3. As a severe chronic-on-subacute slip. These children will have a similar history as those with a subacute slip. However it will be more prolonged. They will also show an external rotation and adduction deformity of the limb. A lateral X-ray will show a severe slip.

4. 'Subclinical slip'. These are only diagnosed retrospectively. They may have had 'growing pains' which stopped an athletic career. They present in adult life with osteoarthritis and in addition the X-rays show flattened femoral heads and slight coxa vara reminiscent of a mild slipped epiphysis.

Treatment (Fig. 19.19)

1. A mild acute slip can be fixed *in situ* with threaded pins. The growth plate will close rapidly and the slip be stabilised.

2. An acute slip can be *gently* manipulated and fixed in its reduced position by threaded pins. This manipulation must be performed within a few hours after the acute slip.

3. A severe chronic slip should be treated initially with traction to relieve spasm. The deformity can then be corrected by a triplane wedge osteotomy (to correct the three components of the deformity).

Complications

The blood supply to the epiphysis is very much in jeopardy and avascular necrosis can occur with catastrophic effects on the hip joint. Manipulation of a slipped epiphysis more than a few hours after the acute event is likely to precipitate avascular necrosis.

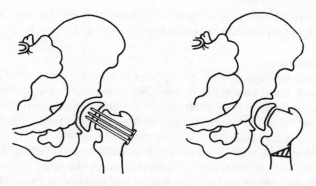

pinning of mild slip   **wedge osteotomy-severe slip**

Fig. 19.19   Treatment of slipped epiphysis.

Another complication described is cartilage necrosis which can lead to severe damage of the hip joint. Its aetiology is unknown, but it appears to be more frequent in Negro children.

The condition is frequently bilateral. There is a 20 per cent chance of the slip occurring on the other side. There is a good case for prophylactic fixation of the other epiphysis to prevent it slipping.

OSTEOARTHRITIS OF THE HIP

This is a condition which occurs frequently in old people. It is a degenerative process characterised by softening and fibrillation of the articular cartilage. In due course this erodes and leaves eburnated bone as the lining of the joint. In addition, the synovial tissue becomes hypertrophic and the capsule becomes thickened and fibrosed. Proliferative changes occur at the margins of the joint forming osteophytes.

Patients present complaining of pain which is felt mainly in the groin. It is also felt in the adjacent buttock and greater trochanter and also down the thigh to the knee and sometimes the shin. This pain is worse particularly on activity and relieved by rest. Classically it is severe on resuming activities after rest.

A patient may also complain of stiffness and limitation of movement in the joint. He will complain of difficulties in dressing, particularly with putting on shoes and socks, in manipulating stairs and getting in and out of cars.

He may also notice an apparent shortening of one leg, which results from an adduction contracture about the hip.

Examination

The patient may walk with a limp, due to either shortening or pain.

He will have limitation of hip joint movement, particularly of flexion, abduction and rotation. In addition, there may be contractures, the commonest of which are a fixed adduction contracture and a fixed flexion deformity of the limb.

There may be wasting of the thigh muscles and also of the glutei. X-rays will show characteristic diminution of the joint space with osteophytes; there maybe sclerosis of the underlying bone. There may be cysts in either the acetabulum or the head of the femur. If the lesion is due to secondary osteoarthritis, there may be characteristic abnormalities of the residual causative condition.

Aetiology

Osteoarthritis is classified as primary (idiopathic) or secondary (Fig. 19.20). A great many cases which used to be considered as primary are now believed to be secondary to some previous condition. The causes of secondary arthritis are:

Trauma. Osteoarthritis rapidly ensues when the joint is severely damaged as result of fractures.

Infection or rheumatoid arthritis. In these conditions, there is primary damage to the synovial fluid and the articular cartilage which it supplies. Osteoarthritic changes rapidly occur secondary to these conditions.

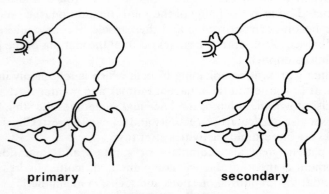

primary   **secondary**

Fig. 19.20   Primary and secondary osteoarthritis.

Perthes' disease, slipped epiphysis and avascular necrosis. In these conditions the head of the femur develops an abnormal shape and incongruity of the joint results.

Conditions such as congenital dislocation of the hip, acetabular dysplasia, and femoral neck anteversion all result in a hip which is unstable. Osteoarthritis occurs in later years.

Treatment

This depends on the severity of the symptoms and the age of the patient. If the symptoms are not severe, the patient may be managed conservatively:

1. Restriction of activities. These patients usually present at or about retiring age and in a great many cases the patient can adapt his lifestyle to suit his disability.

2. The use of a stick in the *opposite* hand. This will afford considerable relief of symptoms by relieving the forces across the hip joint.

3. Judicious use of analgesic and anti-inflammatory drugs. It must be remembered that prolonged use of anti-inflammatory drugs can cause actual deterioration in the condition of the hip joint.

4. Physiotherapy has a part to play in relieving acute symptoms.

If the symptoms are severe, various operative procedures can be undertaken. The most effective and generally used is the total hip replacement (Fig. 19.21c), now a standard and routine operation. In general terms, it consists of replacing the acetabulum by a high density plastic cup and replacing the head of the femur by a metal prosthesis. The components are cemented into place.

Several types of prostheses are in use, and various modes of insertion are used. In 95 per cent of cases dramatically successful results are obtained. However failures do occur and the cause of these failures may be listed:

1. Infection. If infection is established around these prostheses, they work loose and become painful. There is no real alternative but to remove the prosthesis and cement in order to eradicate the infection.

2. Loosening. This can occur when the cement works loose or if the prosthesis itself becomes deformed. A loose prosthesis becomes painful and the symptoms may be severe enough to warrant further operation to replace the prosthesis. This is a much more difficult operation than might be imagined.

3. Fracture of the stem of the prosthesis has been described

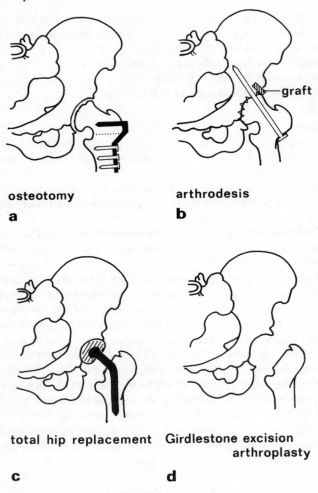

osteotomy

a

arthrodesis

b

—graft

total hip replacement

c

Girdlestone excision
arthroplasty

d

Fig. 19.21   Operative treatment for osteoarthritis.

particularly in heavy and active male patients. Again this patient may present with disabling symptoms and require replacment of the prosthesis.

4. Excessive wear of the prosthesis. This was a problem with earlier models of hip prostheses, but with later models it is not often seen.

5. General complications of the operation include conditions such as deep vein thrombosis and pulmonary embolus.

The procedure has a mortality rate of between 1 and 2 per cent as an older age group is being treated.

Because of these complications, the operation is not usually performed on young patients unless they have a short expectation of life or are very severely disabled. In these patients, other operations can be offered:

1. Osteotomy of the upper end of the femur, usually with firm internal fixation (Fig. 19.21a). This is the modern equivalent of the so-called McMurray's osteotomy. It can afford worthwhile relief of symptoms in patients with osteoarthritis who have a spherical head and a spherical acetabulum. It is contraindicated in more elderly patients.

2. Arthrodesis (Fig. 19.21b). This involves fusion of the hip joint by bone. Technically it is often difficult to achieve and demands either very rigid internal fixation or prolonged immobilisation. This operation is now usually confined to young patients with one hip damaged by either septic arthritis or trauma. This operation is contraindicated in elderly patients (unless special methods are used) and also in patients with disease involving the other hip, the knees, or the back.

3. Excision arthroplasty (Fig. 19.21d). This involves excision of the head and neck of the femur leaving a false flail, fibrous joint (Girdlestone's operation). In fact, when a hip replacement is removed, the patient is left with an excision arthroplasty. These people usually require at least one crutch in order to walk as the hip is unstable, but it is frequently pain-free and mobile. Elderly patients find it very difficult to manage a Girdlestone hip.

RHEUMATOID ARTHRITIS OF THE HIP JOINT

The hip joint is damaged by rheumatoid arthritis as is any other synovial joint in the body. There is proliferation of the synovium and diminution and erosion of the articular cartilage. Eventually secondary osteoarthritic changes ensue. In some patients, the acetabulum appears to soften and the head of the femur 'protrudes' into the pelvis. This condition is called protrusio acetabuli and can be technically very difficult to treat by operation.

If the symptoms are severe enough, these patients warrant operative treatment. The treatment of choice is a total hip replacement. Other forms of operation are rarely satisfactory for treatment of patients with rheumatoid arthritis as so many other joints are involved.

AVASCULAR NECROSIS OF THE HEAD OF THE FEMUR

This condition occurs as a result of gross death of the head of the femur, usually from involvement of its blood supply (see Fig. 7.1, p. 26).

These patients complain of pain in the hip which may be very severe and incapacitating. The hip joint movements are limited and the deformities of fixed flexion and fixed adduction may occur. X-ray will show increased density of the femoral head and in later cases, evidence of collapse of the greater portion of the head.

In early cases in young people, it is reasonable to treat these people conservatively by making them rest as much as possible and reduce weight-bearing by using crutches. Unfortunately in the majority of cases, the disease has progressed so far that such treatment is not worthwhile.

In young patients and in patients in whom the head of the femur has not been deformed, it may be worthwhile drilling out the head of the femur and packing it with cancellous bone grafts. Unfortunately most of the patients seen with this condition are elderly or have severe deformity of the femoral head. In these people, the most generally used operation is the total hip replacement.

There are numerous causes of avascular necrosis:

1. Trauma. This includes subcapital fractures of the neck of the femur (or transcervical fractures in younger patient). Dislocation of the hip.

2. Iatrogenic causes. This includes patients treated with steroids for rheumatoid arthritis or disseminated lupus erythematosus or patients with renal transplants.

3. Alcoholism, liver disease, pancreatitis.

4. Sometimes in pregnancy.

5. Rare causes include sickle-cell anaemia and other haemo-globinopathies, Caisson disease.

6. In a great many cases, the cause is not known and these are classified as idiopathic.

CHAPTER 20

The Knee

HISTORY TAKING

An accurate history is essential to diagnose knee conditions. Certain lesions can be diagnosed on the history alone.

History of injury

The precise mechanism of injury should be elucidated where possible. Usually a rotation or abduction strain is responsible.

The severity of a sports injury is assessed by asking if the patient was able to continue playing or if he had to leave or even be carried off the field.

Patients who have had severe injuries as a result of road traffic accidents can also receive knee injuries. They will often only notice knee symptoms when the effect of other injuries has resolved.

Pain

Pain is usually felt at a specific site in the knee. Any exacerbating or relieving factors are noted.

Swelling

The site and duration of swelling are determined. An effusion occurs above and to each side of the patella.

Sensation of 'letting down'

Sometimes the knee gives way to such an extent that the patient falls. Usually however he only stumbles. This sensation is felt by patients with lesions of the patella who complain of the knee giving way particularly when going down-hill.

Locking
It is important to determine what the patient means by locking. To
orthopaedic surgeons there are three types of locking.
1. 'Pseudo locking' indicates the patient has a spasm of pain and
therefore is unwilling to move the knee. The classical lesion that
causes this is chondromalacia patella.
2. 'Provoked locking' occurs in patients who have meniscus
lesions. The patient will state that he twists on his knee and finds
that following this he is unable to straighten it. Quite often when
performing this sort of manoeuvre, the knee gives way and the
patient falls. When he presents with a locked knee it is found that
there is a definite block to extension of the knee.
3. 'Unprovoked locking' usually occurs with patients with loose
bodies and their locking may occur at any time. Sometimes these
patients are quite unable to extend or flex the knee from the locked
position. This locking is frequently accompanied by the knee giving
way and the patient having a fall. It is often a very distressing
symptom.

EXAMINATION

The examination should be performed with the patient dressed only
in his underpants so that the whole of the lower limb can be
examined. He should be examined both standing and lying down.

With the patient standing
Any obvious deformity of the lower limb such as varus or valgus
deformity (bow legs or knock knees) is noted. The patellae should
be inspected to see if they have normal alignment to the lower
limbs. Some patients with persistent femoral neck anteversion will
stand with the patellae facing inwards ('kissing patellae').
    Any wasting of the quadriceps, effusions or other swellings of the
knee can often be seen better in the standing position. The knee
should be examined from behind in order to see a Baker's cyst or
semimembranosus bursa.

Examination with the patient lying supine
Inspection
The contours of the knee are examined to detect an effusion or
muscle wasting. Wasting of the quadriceps is most easily seen in the

vastus medialis muscle. Any scars, swellings or other abnormalities are noted.

Palpation
The knee is palpated in extension.

The patella is palpated for tenderness around its margins. It is stressed against the femoral condyles – if the patient complains of discomfort he may have chondromalacia. The patella is also stressed laterally out of its groove to detect excessive mobility.

The medial femoral condyle, the lateral femoral condyle, the tibial tubercle and head of fibula are all palpated.

In this position the knee joint is tested for an effusion. One of the easiest ways to detect an effusion in the knee is to press the fluid out of the suprapatellar pouch down behind the patella with one hand. Then keeping the fingers and thumb on each side of the patella, ballotte fluid against them by pressing on the patella with the other hand (Fig. 20.1).

Changes in skin temperatures are noted. The peripheral pulses are examined.

The knee is then palpated when flexed to 90° (Fig. 20.2). The joint line is determined and palpated. The menisci are attached to the joint line. A torn medial meniscus may exhibit tenderness on the joint line medially in front of or behind the medial collateral ligament. The lateral joint line is also palpated for tenderness.

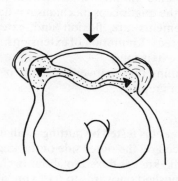

1. **Milk fluid from suprapatellar pouch to patella**

2. **Press on patella and feel transmitted impulse on either side**

Fig. 20.1   Test for effusion in the knee.

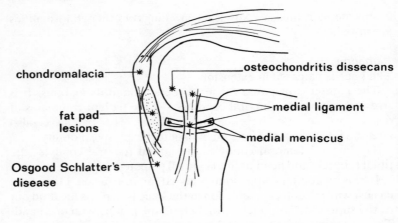

chondromalacia

osteochondritis dissecans

medial ligament

fat pad lesions

medial meniscus

Osgood Schlatter's disease

Fig. 20.2   Points of tenderness in the medial side of knee.

Measurement
The girth of the quadriceps is measured twelve centimetres above the upper pole of the patella and compared with that of the other leg.
The girth of the knee is also measured.

Movements
Both active and passive movements are tested.
Active movements should include straight leg raising which will be impossible if the quadriceps mechanism is damaged.
Passive movements are flexion and extension and can be expressed in degrees. Limitation of extension movements should be noted ('block to extension').
Whilst performing these movements, any pain is noted, and the joint palpated for crepitus.

Ligament stability
The medial ligament is tested by putting a valgus stress on the knee. One hand is placed on the outer side of the knee at the level of the knee joint and the knee is flexed to about twenty degrees and then the lower leg is pushed outwards to try to open up the inner side of the knee. In this position, there is always some movement detectable and it must be compared with the other side (Fig. 20.3).
The reverse procedure is used for the lateral ligament, and again compared to the other side. It is usual to do these tests with the knee

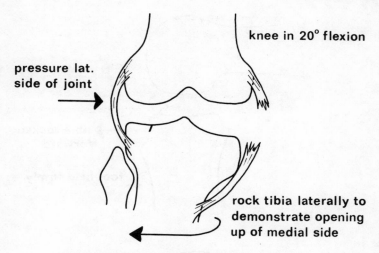

knee in 20° flexion

pressure lat.
side of joint

rock tibia laterally to
demonstrate opening
up of medial side

Fig. 20.3   Testing collateral ligament instability.

flexed to twenty degrees. If the knee is held fully extended, the
posterior cruciate combined with a normal configuration of the joint
will be sufficient to prevent any varus or valgus opening whether the
collateral ligaments are intact or not.

The anterior and posterior cruciate ligaments are tested, the
anterior cruciate by the anterior drawer sign, the posterior cruciate
by the posterior drawer sign. These tests are performed with the
knee flexed to a right angle and the foot held firmly. The anterior
drawer sign consists of drawing the tibia forward on the femoral
condyles. The posterior drawer sign consists of pushing the tibia
backwards on the femoral condyles (Fig. 20.4).

In practice, the pathological anatomy is rather more complicated.
It should also be noted that in the position suggested, if there is a
very lax posterior cruciate, the lower leg will automatically fall back
at the knee joint and pulling forward will produce a very
exaggerated anterior drawer sign; the contour of the knee should be
inspected before performing this manoeuvre.

The McMurray test is a classical test for demonstration of a
meniscus lesion. It is often not positive in patients with a torn
meniscus. In this test, the knee is flexed fully and while slowly
extending it, it is repeatedly externally rotated until about ninety
degrees is reached. In this range from full flexion to ninety degrees,
a torn meniscus may show a positive 'clunking' sensation under the

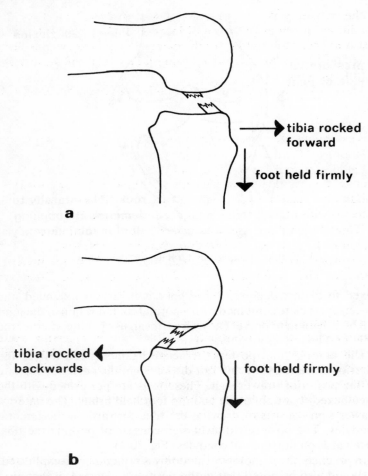

Fig. 20.4   (a) Anterior drawer sign testing anterior cruciate ligament,
(b) posterior drawer sign testing posterior cruciate ligament.

examining hand. In fact a patient may complain of pain on
performing this manoeuvre which is an indication of possible
meniscal damage.

Tests for patella stability
These include the so-called apprehension test where one tries to
dislocate the patella by flexing the knee fully and pressing laterally.

If the patient looks apprehensive it is possible he may have the condition known as recurrent dislocation of the patella. A useful test is to check the stability of the patella in both the extended and flexed position of the knee and see how far lateral it will move in the various positions.

The hip and the ankle on the same side should also be examined.

X-rays

It is essential to X-ray the knee to complete the examination.

Routine AP and lateral X-rays are taken.

Patello-femoral views which show the patella in relation to its groove on the femur are useful. They may be abnormal in conditions such as recurrent subluxation, chondromalacia or osteoarthritis of the patello-femoral compartment.

'Tunnel views' are useful to detect lesions in the intercondylar region such as osteochondritis dissecans or loose bodies.

Arthrograms which involve installation of radiopaque material into the knee are valuable in experienced hands. They are particularly useful in diagnosing meniscus lesions.

Examination under anaesthetic

Examination under anaesthetic is justifiable in assessing acute ligament injuries. These patients are frequently athletes with powerful muscles which are in spasm due to the painful lesion.

It is very difficult to detect any ligament laxity in these patients in the acute stage. In order to make the diagnosis examination of knee ligaments under anaesthesia may be necessary.

Arthroscopy

This involves passing an endoscope through a small incision into the knee joint usually under general anaesthesia. A good view of most of the knee joint except the posterior pouches and an area of the medial compartment can usually be obtained.

In experienced hands this is the most useful investigation to assess knee joint lesions.

SWELLINGS ABOUT THE KNEE JOINT (Fig. 20.5)

An *effusion* into the knee joint occurs frequently after trauma or as a response to inflammation. When present it is most noticeable in the region of the suprapatella pouch and on either side of the patella.

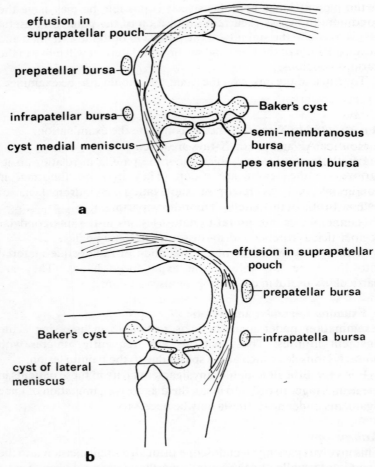

Fig. 20.5   Swellings around the knee, (a) medial side, (b) lateral side.

An effusion can be seen as a convexity above the patella where there is usually a concavity. It can be detected by the 'patella tap' test or by other methods.

Prepatella bursa
This is a bursa directly over the patella and gives the symptoms of 'housemaid's knee'. The lesion is bounded by the margins of the patella. It may become infected following which it may resolve to a

fibrous mass which may be persistently painful. If the lesion causes persistent significant symptoms, it can be simply excised.

Infrapatella bursa
This occurs over the ligamentum patellae just below the patella and has been described as 'clergyman's knee'. It can usually be managed conservatively with rest and a pressure bandage.

Cyst of a meniscus
These occur probably as a result of mucinous degeneration of the centre of the meniscus. There may be an associated tear of the meniscus. Mucinous material passes through the capsule and presents as a cyst. The lateral meniscus cyst is more common.

This lesion may become large. It may also become painful. Characteristically it changes in size according to the position of the joint. If there is persistent pain or symptoms from the associated meniscus tear, the treatment is excision of cyst and a meniscectomy.

Baker's cyst
This is an outpouching of the posterior capsule and is in fact an evidence of effusion of the knee showing itself posteriorly. The treatment is that of the lesion causing the underlying effusion.

Semimembranosus bursa
This is a bursa in relation to the semimembranosus tendon on the posteromedial aspect of the knee. It is in communication with the knee joint and sometimes may become very large with extension among the muscles of the calf.

It is frequently seen in children as a symptomless swelling which usually resolves itself and does not require excision.

In adults it is a manifestation of some other knee pathology such as a meniscus lesion or rheumatoid arthritis. If these lesions are treated, the bursa will frequently disappear. In some patients with rheumatoid arthritis, it may become very large indeed and require excision before the patient obtains relief. Sometimes it may rupture – its fluid will track among the calf muscles causing them to be tender and swollen. This may be mistaken for a deep vein thrombosis.

Certain *bony swellings* occur about the knee joint. In children the most common of these is an osteochondroma. These occur on the inner side of the knee either from the epiphyseal line of the lower end of the femur or from that of the upper end of the tibia.

Patients complain of pain if the lesion is fractured. Sometimes they complain of a clicking sensation which is probably due to the tendons snapping over the lesion.

If it is symptomatic, the swelling should be excised.

Other swellings occur about the knee such as lipomata and ganglia. If a swelling of the knee cannot be diagnosed, it should be explored as very occasionally malignant lesions such as synovial sarcoma may present as a seemingly innocent swelling around the knee joint.

LOOSE BODIES IN THE KNEE JOINT

Loose bodies frequently occur in the knee joint (Fig. 20.6). They are commonly made up of bone and cartilage and once present are maintained in the synovial fluid receiving their nutrient from it. As time passes they are liable to increase in size. They may eventually become trapped in a pouch of synovium or become encapsulated in the fat pad in which case they are unlikely to cause symptoms of locking.

The main complaint of a patient with a loose body is that of locking of the knee. At any time the weight bearing knee may be jammed in one position (usually semi-flexed). This locking is 'unprovoked' as opposed to the locking from which a patient with a meniscus tear will suffer. Sometimes a patient will state that the knee lets him down and he falls. Following the episode of locking, there is often some swelling.

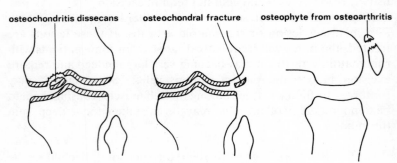

Fig. 20.6　Causes of loose bodies.

On examination there may be wasting of the quadriceps muscle but quite often no other specific physical signs. On other occasions the patient may actually point out to the examiner the presence of a loose body, which can be felt through the capsule of the joint as a mobile nodule. Most loose bodies are visible on X-ray. Some, however, are made entirely of cartilage and these are not seen.

Osteochondritis dissecans

This is frequently seen in adolescents and children. It is assumed that for some reason the blood supply of this area of bone and cartilage is lost and in due course it becomes shed into the joint. The patients will complain initially of a feeling of weakness and repeated sensation of letting down and an effusion in the knee. When the lesion is shed into the joint they will complain of unprovoked locking characteristic of a loose body.

X-ray may show the lesion outlined by an area of radiolucency. If a loose body has been shed in the joint, it will be apparent on X-ray if sufficient views are taken.

If the lesion is not separated it may be treated by rest in a plaster cylinder.

If this fails after two or three months, the lesion may be repaired with cortical grafts taken from the tibia., These it is hoped will permit revascularisation of the lesion and permit its reattachment. However if the lesion is separated or just hinging, it is probably best to excise it, and leave an irregular area to fill (in due course) with fibro-cartilage. Such patients may develop osteoarthritic changes in the knees at a later date on account of the incongruity of the joint.

Osteochondral fractures

The knee joint may be subjected to a sheer stress. In which case, it is quite possible for a portion of cartilage with a small piece of the underlying bone to be sheered off into the knee joint. This will maintain itself in the synovial fluid as a loose body. Furthermore as it contains predominantly cartilage it will not be easily seen on X-ray. These patients will give a very definite history of injury followed by haemarthrosis into the knee. After the injury has resolved, they may complain of repeated episodes of locking or of the knee giving way. These osteochondral fracture lesions are relatively common and a patient with such symptoms and a normal X-ray should be investigated to exclude the possibility of an osteochondral fracture persisting as a loose body. The treatment is to remove the loose fragment.

Osteoarthritis

Patients with osteoarthritis of the knee may produce loose bodies, probably from breaking off of osteophytes. These are quite common X-ray findings. The loose bodies may be attached to the synovium and will therefore not cause significant symptoms of locking. Only if a patient with osteoarthritis has definite episodes of locking should the so-called 'loose body' be removed.

Osteochondromatosis

The synovial membrane forms cartilage and bony swellings in great numbers. In the well developed case, the whole suprapatellar pouch may feel like a bag of marbles. These may well cause symptoms of locking. If the locking is severe, the joint should be explored and the loose bodies removed. In order to prevent further recurrences, a synovectomy of the joint should be performed.

MENISCUS LESIONS IN THE KNEE

The menisci are made of fibrocartilage. They are avascular and when torn will probably not heal. Tears are produced by a rotation force on the flexed weight bearing knee.

In the young person, the meniscus is strong. In the older patient it becomes degenerate and there may be an area of mucinous degeneration in the centre of the meniscus. The degenerate meniscus of an older patient is more easily torn and is subject to a different type of tear than the meniscus of a young patient (Fig. 20.7).

Medial meniscus

In young patients, the tear is a result of a rotational force, which occurs commonly with sporting injuries. The patient can often give a fairly precise history of the mechanism. He will complain of sudden severe pain on the side of the knee affected, it may lock and the pain is such that he has to stop playing. Over the succeeding few hours the knee becomes swollen. The symptoms may subside but are liable to recur more easily with subsequent twisting motion applied to the knee.

An older patient will complain of twisting the knee whilst kneeling or squatting and developing a sudden pain in the knee which is followed by swelling. The pain and swelling are persistent and they may complain of a clicking sensation in the knee.

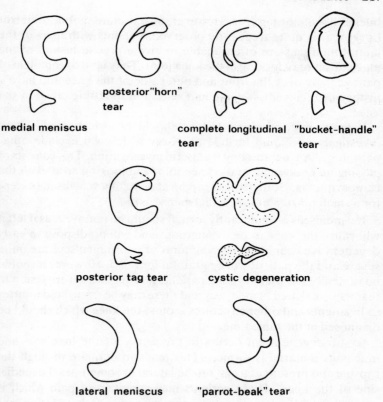

Fig. 20.7   Meniscus lesions.

In young patients, a longitudinal tear is produced and it is visualised as starting in the posterior horn of the meniscus and extending anteriorly. When the patient gives a history of locking, the central torn portion dislocates into the centre of the joint forming the so-called 'bucket handle'. This is enough to stop full extension of the knee. In older patients, a horizontal tear is usually produced and it is again seen in the posterior horn usually as a horizontal tag; however, any portion of the meniscus may be affected.

Lateral meniscus

The lateral meniscus is affected less frequently than the medial meniscus. It may be torn in a similar manner producing either a bucket handle or tag tear. However, as it is more mobile a 'parrot beak' tear is quite frequently observed. Patients with tears of the lateral meniscus are often unable to give a precise history of the mechanism or of locking in the knee joint. They tend to complain of pain vaguely over the front and outer side of the knee and have a history of recurrent swelling and sensation of letting down in the knee.

Patients with meniscus lesions should be investigated. These investigations should include an X-ray which will exclude other pathology. An arthroscopy is a useful investigation. This consists of passing an endoscope in the knee joint and looking around all the compartments. Both menisci can be almost fully visualised (except for a small portion of the medial meniscus).

If a meniscus is significantly torn, it should be removed, as if left it will cause the knee to be incongruous and will predispose to early degenerative changes. The symptoms of a torn meniscus are quite severe and the patient will be grateful for relief. However it should be remembered that in young patients it requires a severe lesion to tear a normal medial meniscus and there may be associated injuries to ligaments and other structures around the knee which should be diagnosed at the same time.

Cystic degeneration occurs in the centre of the meniscus and mucinous material is formed. This tends to herniate through the capsule and present as a cyst on the lateral or sometimes the medial side of the knee. These patients may complain of pain which is associated with a degenerative or torn meniscus. If these lesions are symptomatic they should be treated by excision of the cyst and the underlying meniscus.

In children, particularly on the lateral side, the meniscus may form abnormally; instead of presenting a normal semilunar configuration it presents as a disc. Patients with discoid menisci will complain of a significant 'clunk' on movements of the knee and if this is persistently painful and causing discomfort, a meniscectomy may be performed to remove it.

KNEE LIGAMENT INSTABILITY

The stability of the knee joint depends on its capsule and associated ligaments. The normal movements of the knee are flexion and extension. Full extension is accompanied by medial rotation of the femur on the tibia (so-called 'screw home' movement). This last rotation is dependent upon the normal functioning of both anterior and posterior cruciate ligaments.

After injury the ligaments may be completely disrupted or merely stretched.

Treatment of knee ligament injuries is often imperfect and patients are left with some laxity of either the collateral or cruciate ligaments or both.

These patients will complain of a sensation of giving way of the knee when this particular ligament is stressed. This may be followed by swelling and associated pain. Often these symptoms are only such as to preclude partaking of a particular sporting activity. However they may be sufficient to interfere with ordinary walking or running.

Certain ligament syndromes are described.

Medial complex injuries
This is usually due to damage of the medial ligament and there may be associated damage of the medial meniscus and of the anterior cruciate ligament (O'Donoghue's triad) (Fig. 20.8).

On examination these patients will show definite valgus laxity when stressing the medial ligament complex and they may also have a positive anterior drawer sign particularly with the foot in external rotation. The function of these patients' knees can be improved by operation to strengthen the medial complex of ligaments. The tendon most frequently used to strengthen them is the semi-tendinosus.

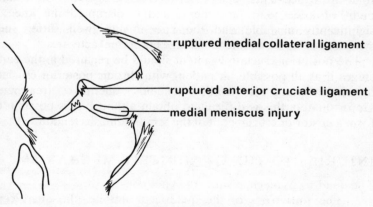

ruptured medial collateral ligament

ruptured anterior cruciate ligament
medial meniscus injury

Fig. 20.8   Abduction injuries.

Lateral complex injuries
These are less frequent, and sometimes occur after motor vehicle accidents. The lateral complex includes the lateral ligament and also the insertion of the fascia lata to the upper end of the tibia. These patients will have similar symptoms but, unless they are athletes, the injuries will not be severe enough to require operative treatment.

Rotary instability
This is usually associated with either rupture or stretching of the anterior cruciate ligament in association with either the medial or lateral ligament complexes. Various types of rotary instability are described. Those most frequently seen are antero-medial rotary instability and antero-lateral rotary instability in association with injuries to the medial and lateral ligament complexes respectively.

These patients complain of a sensation of giving way after stressing the ligaments concerned. Unless they are athletes the symptoms can usually be controlled by building up of the quadriceps muscle to supplement the anterior cruciate dysfunction. However if they are involved in contact sports, this is frequently not sufficient and various operations have been devised to assist this sort of instability with equally varying results.

Posterior cruciate ligament
Injuries to the posterior cruciate ligament (see Fig. 12.2, p. 67) may be associated with injuries to the other collateral ligaments of the knee. These injuries occur as a result of severe trauma such as road traffic accidents. The posterior cruciate ligament is the main pivot of knee joint movement, and if disrupted the knee is significantly unstable and the patient may well suffer such symptoms as to be unable to manage his normal activities.

The posterior cruciate ligament should be repaired in the early stages if at all possible. A patient with chronic posterior cruciate ligament injury frequently demands operative treatment. Unfortunately this is difficult to obtain although it is possible to form a posterior cruciate out of the semitendinosus tendon.

INJURIES TO THE QUADRICEPS MECHANISM

The quadriceps mechanism of the knee consists of:
1. The four parts of the quadriceps muscle, the quadriceps expansion and its attachment to the patella.

2. The patella and its associated retinaculum.
3. The ligamentum patellae.
4. The tibial tuberosity.

The quadriceps mechanism can be injured by direct or indirect violence.

By direct violence. The best example of this is the 'dashboard' injury to the occupant of a motor vehicle involved in an accident which produces a direct fracture of the patella. This tends to be a comminuted fracture which is not necessarily widely separated.

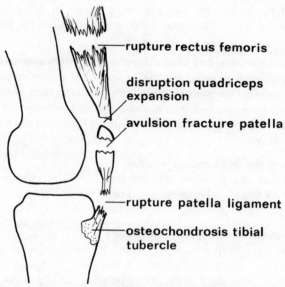

rupture rectus femoris

disruption quadriceps expansion

avulsion fracture patella

rupture patella ligament

osteochondrosis tibial tubercle

Fig. 20.9   Injuries to the quadriceps mechanism.

Indirect violence injuries are due to a sudden contracture of the quadriceps muscle against fixed resistance. This will produce a series of injuries (Fig. 20.9).

Rupture of rectus femoris
Rupture of the rectus femoris is found on occasions in young athletes after excessive exertion. The patient presents with a swelling in the muscle. This is fairly easily repaired if the patient presents early and the lesion is diagnosed. Even if it is not repaired function is still very good if it is managed conservatively.

Rupture of the quadriceps expansion

This occurs fairly frequently in elderly people. The classical mechanism is that the patient stumbles against the curb as he is walking. The quadriceps contracts and avulses itself from its attachment to the patella.

This is frequently difficult to diagnose as the X-ray shows no fracture. There is considerable swelling. There is a palpable gap just above the patella and the patient will be unable to perform an active straight leg raise.

It is essential that this is diagnosed as it requires operative repair followed by immobilisation for some weeks in order to restore adequate function of the quadriceps and to stabilise the knee.

Fracture of the patella

Fractures due to this type of injury are usually transverse and the fragments are separated by the action of the quadriceps. These patients require operative repair, fixing the fracture; if the patella fracture is comminuted it is excised and the patellar retinaculum repaired. The knee must be immobilised for some time following this operation.

Rupture of the ligamentum patellae

The ligamentum patellae rupture can occur, as can an avulsion fracture of the tibial tuberosity. These lesions require operative repair.

Osteochondrosis of the tibial tuberosity

Over-use injuries in young people produce osteochondrosis of the tibial tubercle (Osgood Schlatter's disease). This occurs in early adolescence. Patients complain of a painful swelling in the region of the tibial tubercle.

The treatment is rest and restriction of activities. If the symptoms persist, they will usually resolve if the knee is immobilised in a plaster cylinder. Very occasionally a persistent sequestrum forms at the site of the lesion which may cause symptoms severe enough to require removal.

LESIONS OF THE PATELLA

Recurrent dislocation of the patella (Fig. 20.10)

The patella dislocates laterally. Having once dislocated, episodes of dislocation frequently recur.

The patella usually dislocates in the flexed position of the knee. The patient is unable to straighten the knee. If the knee is straightened, then the patella will usually reduce itself. These patients may complain of locking because they find they are unable to straighten the knee, and then they can suddenly do so as the patella clicks back into position.

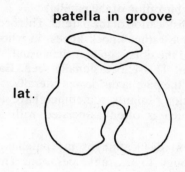

patella in groove

lat.

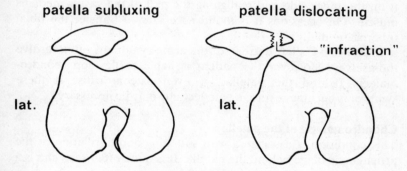

patella subluxing

lat.

patella dislocating

"infraction"

lat.

Fig. 20.10   Dislocating patella.

In addition to this the patient complains of persistent sensation of the knee feeling weak and having a tendency to give way. They complain occasionally of pain and weakness particularly on going downstairs or downhill.

On examination there is often wasting of the quadriceps muscle, particularly the vastus medialis. The patella is very mobile and can be subluxed or even dislocated on examination. X-ray of the knee should include a patello-femoral view, and this may show a small infraction caused by the episodes of dislocation. It may also show malalignment of the patella in its groove on the lower end of the femur.

Recurrent dislocation of the patella can be classified as:

Post-traumatic. This occurs in young athletes, girls as well as boys. There is often a definite history of an initial injury followed by repeated episodes of dislocation or even of persistent weakness (so-called recurrent-subluxation of the patella).

Classical recurrent dislocation of the patella. This occurs in young ladies who usually have rather knock knees, in whom the angle between the femur and the tibia is greater than usual.

Habitual dislocation. This is occasionally seen. Each time the patient flexes his knee the patella dislocates laterally.

Congenital dislocation. Infants sometimes have a very small dislocated patella which is often associated with knee flexion deformity.

Patients with recurrent dislocation of the patella usually have symptoms severe enough to warrant operation. This operation usually consists of releasing the patella on the outer side and reefing it on the inner side and realigning the pull of the vastus medialis muscle. On occasions it is found necessary to transfer the tibial tubercle medially.

If the lesion is left untreated, the acute symptoms often resolve themselves. However the patient is liable to develop chondromalacia behind the patella, or even osteoarthritis. If these symptoms become severe, a patellectomy may be necessary.

Chondromalacia of the patella

This condition is associated with softening and fibrillation of the articular cartilage behind the patella. It is quite often seen and is a frequent cause of symptoms about the knee.

It may be caused by:

Trauma. Following direct violence such as dashboard injuries of road traffic accidents.

In association with recurrent dislocation or subluxation of the patella, this is probably one of the commonest causes.

Idiopathic. The patients will complain of aching in the knee after exercise and after going up and particularly down hill. This pain and aching may be associated with an effusion. There is also a sensation of the knee giving way. The condition may be associated with the syndrome of recurrent dislocation or subluxation of the patella.

On examination, these patients frequently have wasting of the quadriceps muscle. Stressing the patella produces pain and often crepitus.

An X-ray should be taken and is frequently normal. The patello-femoral view may show some narrowing between the patella and the femur, and a malalignment of the patella in the patello-femoral groove. Sometimes cystic changes are seen in the patella adjacent to the joint space.

An arthroscopy is a useful investigation as it is possible to determine how much of the patella is subject to chondromalacia and how severe it is.

These patients are usually difficult to treat. Many cases can be treated by reduction of activities, in particular those which are liable to put excessive pressure on the patella like sprinting, long jumping and bicycle racing.

More severe cases can sometimes be relieved by operation. That which is frequently used is to release the patella on the outer side and reef it on the inner side. This may be accompanied by shaving the area of chondromalacia.

Patients with severe chondromalacia causing persistent symptoms would benefit from a patellectomy.

OSTEOARTHRITIS OF THE KNEE

The knee joint is very frequently affected by osteoarthritis. It is often found in old people, particularly those who are overweight. In the majority there is no specific cause for the condition.

However, there are certain conditions which will predispose to osteoarthritis of the knees and these are:

Conditions which will cause damage to the actual joint surfaces, such as fractures, rheumatoid and septic arthritis and also loose fragments such as loose bodies or torn menisci.

Lesions such as ligament injuries which cause the knee to be unstable.

Lesions which result in malalignment of the knee such as bow legs, knock knees or subluxation of the patella.

The knee can be considered as having three main compartments. These are the patello-femoral, medial tibio-femoral, and the lateral tibio-femoral compartments. In a great many patients, all three compartments are affected by osteoarthritis, but in some, only one or two compartments are involved.

Patients will complain predominantly of pain in the knee. They will also have episodes of swelling. They may complain of a feeling of instability. This feeling of instability is more marked when going up or down hill.

On examination these patients will show quadriceps wasting. There may be some peri-articular thickening of the soft tissues around the knee. There may be an effusion. Knee movements will be limited and crepitus can be felt on moving the knee. Malalignment may be obvious. There may be associated instability.

X-rays will show narrowing of the joint space in the compartment affected with osteophytes at the margins, sharpening of the tibial spines, and there will be underlying sclerosis.

Treatment
The majority of patients can be managed conservatively. Many patients have osteoarthritic changes in the knee joint with no symptoms. An episode such as minor trauma seems to trigger off the symptoms which can be self-limiting and amenable to simple treatment:

1. Anti-inflammatory drugs such as indomethacin and Isobrufen can be invaluable in these acute episodes.

2. Patients should be advised to reduce activities temporarily in any case. Some patients tend to lead an active sporting life rather longer than they should and these should be advised to desist.

3. Pressure bandages, in particular a horse shoe pad and bandage, can afford great relief. Bracing of the knee is not always very effective.

4. Physiotherapy is of value in building up the quadriceps muscle. If this is strong and active the knee is made much more stable. Other physiotherapy treatment, such as heat and ultrasound, is of value.

5. These patients are frequently over-weight and should be advised to lose weight. If they can do so, their symptoms may be dramatically relieved.

Operative treatment
If the patello-femoral compartment only is involved a *patellectomy* may be indicated. Unfortunately most patients who have damage of the patello-femoral compartment also have damage of the other compartments of the knee.

If either the medial or lateral tibio-femoral compartment is

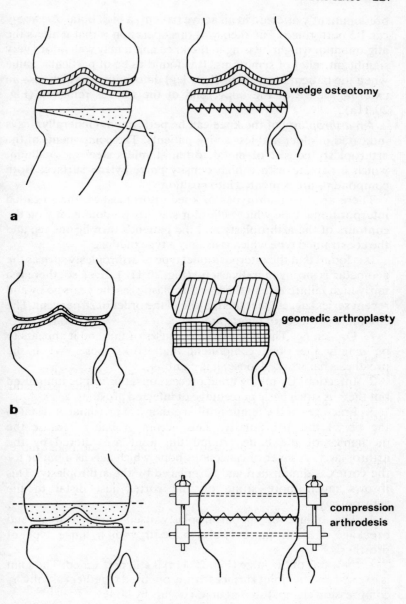

a   wedge osteotomy

b   geomedic arthroplasty

c   compression arthrodesis

Fig. 20.11   Treatment for osteoarthritis in the knee.

predominantly affected in an active patient, a high tibial *osteotomy* can be performed. The theory of this operation is that it alters the alignment of weight bearing in the knee and it may well afford very significant relief of symptoms. It is found to be of particular value when the patient has a varus (bow leg) deformity, in which case an external wedge of the upper end of the tibia is removed (Fig. 20.11a).

An *arthroplasty* of the knee can be performed. Generally this is indicated in older and less active patients. The components of the arthroplasty consist of metal, often stainless steel or vitallium, which articulate with a high density polyethylene surface. Both components are cemented into position.

There are two main types of knee arthroplasties, the so-called interpositional type which relies for stability predominantly on the contours of the arthroplasty and the patient's own ligaments; and the constrained type which is usually a type of hinge.

It is found that the interpositional type of arthroplasty such as the geomedic is most generally useful (Fig. 20.11b). Even so, there is a fairly high failure rate of these arthroplasties as the years go by and recent series suggest that this may be of the order of 20 per cent. The commonest causes of failure are:

1. Loosening. There are various causes of this and it appears to be mainly the tibial component that works loose. When the prosthesis has worked loose, it is painful.

2. Infection. By taking great precautions, this can be minimised but there is still a basic percentage of infected prostheses.

3. Fractures of the femur or tibia either just proximal or distal to the tip of the arthroplasty. This occurs probably because the mechanics of the bone around the joint are altered by the arthroplasty. A layer of cancellous bone which acts as a buffer for the cortex is diminished and is replaced by the arthroplasty. This throws much more strain on the cortex just distal to the arthroplasty.

4. The failure of the arthroplasty itself through wear and breakage. This is more likely to occur with a hinge type of prosthesis.

Arthrodesis of the knee (Fig. 20.11c) is still performed. The joint is excised and the joint surfaces firmly opposed together (usually by compression clamps) so that union occurs by bone.

This provides a stable knee which is painless. However it does have disadvantages in that it throws more strain on the other joints, and also a stiff knee is a considerable encumbrance particularly when sitting, travelling by car and walking up and down steps.

RHEUMATOID ARTHRITIS OF THE KNEE

As with all other joints, the knee is affected in rheumatoid arthritis (see Fig. 11.1, p. 57). In some patients it may be the only joint affected which makes the diagnosis difficult.

In the acute stage, the patient presents with an acute painful effusion. The X-ray may be normal. Aspiration and temporary immobilisation of the knee may afford satisfactory relief of symptoms and also help with the diagnosis.

The patient may have persistent synovial thickening and effusions. She will present with a persistently painful swollen knee. The knee will be stable on stressing and there will be over ninety degrees of flexion movement. The X-ray will show a good joint space. Such a knee would benefit from a synovectomy (an operation to remove as much of the damaged synovium inside the knee joint as possible).

In the later stages of the disease, the knee is badly disorganised. It may be very painful and very unstable due to stretching of the ligaments and collapse of the underlying bone; surgery may be required because of this painful instability. It may be practically ankylosed due to loss of all the articular cartilage and formation of fibrous adhesions inside the joint. These knees are also very painful and may require surgical treatment.

At this stage surgery consists of a replacement arthroplasty. If the knee is reasonably stable it can be an interpositional type. If it is very unstable, then a constrained type of arthroplasty should be considered. Arthrodesis of the knee may be indicated but unfortunately patients with rheumatoid arthritis may have so many other joints involved that they find it difficult to manage with an arthrodesed knee.

SEPTIC ARTHRITIS OF THE KNEE

Septic arthritis occurs in the knee as frequently as any other joint. It is found predominantly in the young patient and in the very old. In the very young patient the joint is hot, swollen and exquisitely painful. The diagnosis is confirmed by aspiration of the purulent fluid. Treatment consists of aspirations which are repeated as necessary. The joint is immobilised with a back slab and relevant antibiotics are given. If the infection is persistent, it may be necessary to perform a formal arthrotomy of the knee joint.

In the very old patient, the disease is slightly different and these patients may present with an effusion and general malaise. The joint may be slightly warm, but not particularly painful. The diagnosis is made by aspirating the swollen joint. This diagnosis must be considered in any geriatric patient because if the condition persists the joint will be gradually destroyed and the patient become more and more incapacitated.

PSEUDO GOUT OF THE KNEE

This is a condition where there is a deposition of calcium pyrophosphate crystals in joints. The knee is the commonest joint affected. The patient suffers an acute exacerbation of pain and swelling in the knee with all the appearance of septic arthritis except there is only a low grade temperature. X-ray may show the menisci to be outlined in calcification. Aspiration of the knee will permit the diagnosis to be made. The fluid which is extracted should be examined under polarised light for monorefrigent crystals which are diagnostic of the condition. Treatment is by aspiration and immobilisation in the acute phase and the condition rapidly resolves with treatment with phenylbutazone. These patients are of course liable to recurrences of this condition.

GENU VARUM (bow legs)

In children
Bow legs (Fig. 20.12a) are commonly seen in rather over-weight children in the first two years of life. Almost always these correct themselves without treatment. Very occasionally treatment with plaster casts or splints is indicated.

Occasionally bow legs is a manifestation of rickets. Renal rickets is more common than nutritional rickets in Western countries at the present time. These children may present with marked bow legs and the diagnosis is made on X-ray and by biochemical tests. Severe bowing of the legs may need correction by a tibial osteotomy.

A progressive deformity known as Blount's disease may occur in Negro children. They have a progressively increasing varus deformity of their knees and X-ray shows an abnormality of the

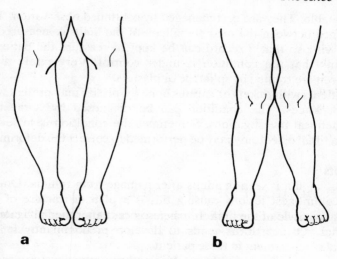

Fig. 20.12 (a) Genu varum, (b) genu valgum.

medial side of the upper tibial epiphysis. These children always require treatment to correct the deformity. Frequently a tibial osteotomy is necessary.

Adults
Patients frequently develop osteoarthritis in the medial compartment of their knees. These people often have a varus deformity. If the medial compartment is the area predominantly affected, the symptoms may be relieved by an upper tibial osteotomy.

Patients who have had a previous medial meniscectomy can develop a varus deformity of their knees in later life and this is associated with degenerative changes occurring in the knee. Fairly marked deformities of the knee are seen in patients with Paget's disease.

GENU VALGUM (knock knees)

In children
Knock knees (Fig. 20.12b) are frequently seen in young children. It appears to be associated with valgus heels and internally rotated lower limbs. This condition usually corrects without treatment. By the time the child is aged six or seven, the condition is barely

noticeable. They are best managed by continued observation. The distance between the medial malleoli of the limbs is measured at each visit so that a record can be kept to reassure the patient's parents that the condition is under control. Very rarely these children are treated by splintage or plasters.

Patients with rickets or various bone dysplasias may present with knock knees. The condition can be diagnosed by X-ray and biochemical investigations. Sometimes the condition is so severe that a tibial osteotomy may be performed to correct the deformity.

Adults

Genu valgum is seen in adults after damage from trauma. One of the commonest lesions causing this is a plateau fracture of the lateral condyle of the tibia. It may also occur after medial ligament injuries. Osteoarthritis tends to develop predominantly in the lateral compartment in these patients.

Patients with severe rheumatoid arthritis can develop grossly valgus and unstable knees. Such knees are very difficult to treat and are best managed with a constrained type of total knee prosthesis.

GENU RECURVATUM (back knee)

There is a considerable variation in the degree of hyperextension which occurs in people's knees. A normal person may have a back knee of nearly ten degrees without symptoms.

An abnormal degree of back knee is seen in patients with generalised joint laxity and in such people no treatment is indicated. This generalised laxity can also be seen by examining the elbows and the metacarpophalangeal joints of the fingers. In both cases, an abnormal amount of hyperextension can be elicited.

A severe degree of back knee is sometimes seen in patients who have had damage to the epiphysis of the upper end of the tibia. The tibial tubercle in the child is developed from the epiphysis of the upper end of the tibia. Damage to the tibial tubercle can cause growth to cease in the anterior portion and as a result a back knee will develop inevitably in future years. Sometimes this deformity is so severe that a tibial osteotomy is required to correct it. A back knee can be seen in patients who have laxity of the posterior capsule and posterior cruciate ligaments after trauma. It is also sometimes seen in patients who have an equinus deformity of the foot. In order to make the foot plantigrade they have to hyperextend the knee.

FIXED FLEXION DEFORMITY

A fixed flexion deformity can occur in neurological conditions and also in a knee which has been damaged by osteoarthritis or rheumatoid arthritis.

It causes a considerable amount of disability because it alters the mechanical efficiency of the weight bearing knee. A knee with a fixed flexion deformity puts undue strain on the quadriceps mechanism and these patients find great difficulty in prolonged standing and balancing.

It is difficult to correct this deformity, but the symptoms are so much improved by even a partial correction that it is worth attempting. Even bedridden patients with a severe fixed flexion deformity of the knees will be made very much easier to nurse if the knees can be straightened.

CHAPTER 21

Foot and Ankle

The foot provides a stable platform for weight bearing. This platform is not only stable, it is mobile. This mobility allows for variations in ground surface and also allows for the rotation movements of the lower limb which occur in normal walking.

The normal weight bearing areas of the foot are the metatarsal heads and the posterior portion of the calcaneus.

The shape of the foot and the relation of these weight bearing areas to each other depends on the bones, the joints and ligaments and the plantar fascia. Muscle activity is not required to maintain the arch of the foot in standing.

The alterations required to permit even weight bearing by the foot are subserved by movements of the subtalar joint (which acts as an oblique hinge). Reciprocal movements occur at the joints between the tarsal bones and the metatarsals to permit realignment of the metatarsal heads.

Abnormalities in the weight bearing areas of the foot can produce symptoms severe enough to require treatment.

However, if the foot is rigid, but in a normal position, the patient can walk quite adequately on a flat regular surface provided he has some residual ankle movement. Similarly, a patient with a rigid ankle can manage quite adequately provided there is some residual mobility in the foot.

Footwear can be adapted to accommodate some degree of deformity; e.g. an equinus deformity can be alleviated by providing a raised heel. Severe degrees of deformity in the foot demand operative treatment. The ankle and subtalar joints are weight bearing joints. Degenerative changes in these joints can produce severe symptoms which demand treatment.

The main function of footwear would appear to be to protect the foot against trauma, climate and infection. However, footwear can cause deformities in children as occurred in Chinese girls in the past. Present-day Australian school shoes frequently have hard rigid uppers and composition soles; when these are worn by children who have run barefoot during the summer holidays, numerous local problems occur. When adults wear shoes with pointed toes which cramp the forefoot, combined with high heels with no platform, symptoms of metatarsalgia inevitably occur.

HISTORY TAKING

Symptoms in the foot and ankle usually have a local cause. The common symptoms complained of are:

Pain
Site of the pain is important as it may well indicate the site of the lesion. Exacerbating factors should be noted. The pain may well be related to deformities such as a bunion or to certain particular activities.

Deformities
These will often be described by the patient quite adequately but in non-medical terms.

Swelling
Swelling is often described as occurring around the ankle or foot. Remember that there are many causes of generalised swelling of the ankle and the feet and both lower limbs must be examined.

Any history of injury should be noted.

EXAMINATION

The patient should be examined with both lower limbs fully exposed. He should be examined first standing and then sitting with the foot free. Finally the shoes should be inspected.

Examination with the patient standing

Inspection
The feet and ankles are inspected for any localised swelling. Deformities are noted, particularly in the toes, in the longitudinal

arch and in the overall shape of the foot. The foot should also be examined from behind to see the shape of the heel (Fig. 21.1).

The normal foot is plantigrade (at right angles to the leg) (Fig. 21.2a).

Equinus foot (Fig 21.2b) is one with a fixed flexion deformity of the foot. The patient may stand with his heel raised from the ground.

Calcaneus foot (Fig. 21.2c) is one with a fixed dorsi flexion deformity so the forefoot cannot be placed on the ground and most of the weight is taken on the heel.

Abnormalities of the longitudinal arch are described.

Flat foot (pes planus) (Fig. 21.2e). In such a foot, the longitudinal

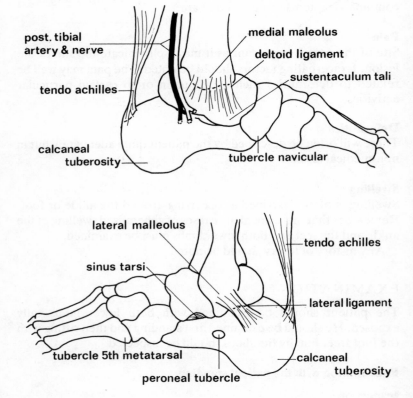

Fig. 21.1   Landmarks of the foot and ankle, (a) medial side, (b) lateral side.

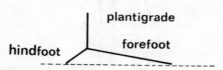

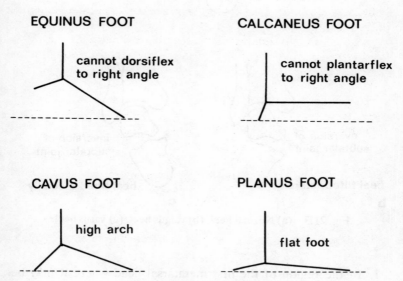

Fig. 21.2 Foot deformities.

arch is flattened more than usual. It may often be associated with a
heel that points outwards (valgus heel).

Cavus foot (Fig. 21.2d). This means that the foot has a raised
longitudinal arch. Patients with this condition present in childhood
or adolescence and should be carefully investigated, as the lesion
may have a neurological cause.

Valgus heel (Fig. 21.3b). This is associated with flat foot, but it is
also seen with abnormalities of the subtalar joint or the calcaneus.

Varus heel (Fig. 21.3c) points inwards. It is seen with numerous
other foot deformities and is useful indicator of their correction.

Exostosis is a term used for a bony prominence of the foot. These
are seen:

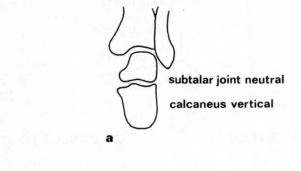

subtalar joint neutral

calcaneus vertical

a

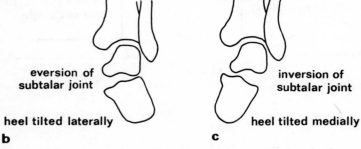

eversion of
subtalar joint

inversion of
subtalar joint

heel tilted laterally

heel tilted medially

b

c

Fig. 21.3   (a) Normal heel, (b) valgus heel, (c) varus heel.

1. In the region of the first metatarsal head where it may be associated with a bunion.

2. A bunionette occurs on the outer side of the head of the fifth metatarsal. The base of the fifth metatarsal may be unduly prominent and cause pain from shoe pressure.

3. The joint of the first metatarsal with the medial cuneiform may be the site of an exostosis, causing symptoms from shoe pressure.

4. The postero-lateral aspect of the calcaneus may be the site of a bony prominence which will cause pain from shoe pressure.

All the above lesions may be found in children and usually can be relieved by advice as to wearing comfortable shoes. On occasions, the symptoms are so persistent that the exostosis has to be removed.

Examination with the patient sitting

Patients should then be examined with the legs hanging free over the side of the examination couch.

Palpation

Palpation for tender areas (Fig. 21.4) may include:

The medial and lateral malleoli and the ankle joint.

Posteriorly over the tendo achilles, and its attachment to the calcaneus.

Beneath the calcaneus at the site of the attachment to the plantar fascia.

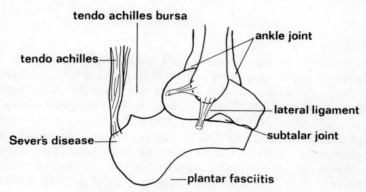

tendo achilles bursa

ankle joint

tendo achilles

lateral ligament

Sever's disease

subtalar joint

plantar fasciitis

Fig. 21.4   Tender areas around the heel.

The sinus tarsi should be palpated just anterior to the lateral malleolus – tenderness here indicates a lesion of the subtalar joint.

The site of the midtarsal joint should be palpated.

The metatarsophalangeal joints and the metatarsal heads.

Callosities

These are frequently painful and found in areas of undue pressure.

In particular, callosities on the sole of the foot should be examined and are frequently found to be abnormal in the region of the metatarsal heads.

Movement

Movement of the various joints is noted and compared with the normal foot and ankle. Active movements are noted first and then passive movements.

The ankle joint involves dorsiflexion and plantar flexion movements (Fig. 21.5). The normal range of dorsiflexion is ten or

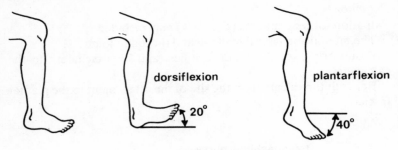

Fig. 21.5　Ankle movements.

even twenty degrees above a right angle. The normal range of plantar flexion is some thirty or forty degrees below the right angle.

The movements at the subtalar joint usually have to be determined passively. This is done by holding the patient's leg in one hand and rotating the heel and foot with the other into inversion and eversion (Fig. 21.6). The axis of this rotation passes from the lateral aspect of the heel to the inner side of the head of the talus.

Movements of the midtarsal joint can also only be determined passively. The heel is steadied with one hand and the forefoot rotated with the other (Fig. 21.7).

The movement of the toes are determined actively and passively, in particular, the movements of the metatarsophalangeal joint of

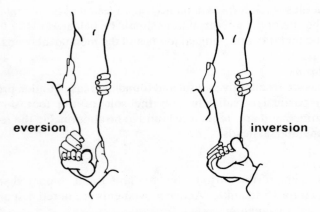

move foot & heel passively

Fig. 21.6　Movements at the subtalar joint.

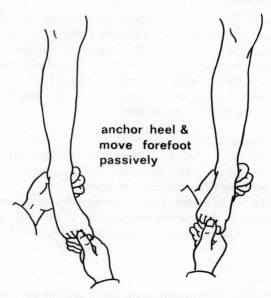

anchor heel &
move forefoot
passively

Fig. 21.7 Movement at the midtarsal joint.

the big toe are noted. There is a condition called hallux rigidus in which the movement of the big toe is limited.

Examination with the patient prone
The patient is then examined prone on the couch and in this position the tendo achilles, the back of the ankle and the heel can be fully examined.

The shoes are then inspected for any excessive wear, either in the uppers or in the soles. The thickness and rigidity of the soles is determined. The material of which the uppers is made is noted. The height and stability of the heel and also the heel platform is noted to see whether it is satisfactory.

TOE ABNORMALITIES

Curly toes
This deformity is frequently seen in children. One or more of the minor toes may be curved medially at the distal interphalangeal joint.

The majority of patients require no treatment as they have no symptoms and the deformity gradually disappears. However some children have persistent symptoms in particular if the toe underlies an adjacent toe, and develops symptoms from shoe pressure.

Treatment by strapping is often advised but is of doubtful value. An operation may be performed to transfer the long flexor tendon of the toe to its extensor expansion.

Mallet deformity

The patients have a flexion deformity of the distal interphalangeal joint of a minor toe. This frequently causes symptoms from shoe pressure over the tip of the distal phalanx.

In a child, the deformity can be corrected by transferring the long flexor tendon to the extensor expansion. In an adult, it is best to arthrodese the distal interphalangeal joint of the toe in the correct position.

Hammer toes

This deformity is frequently seen in adolescents and young adults. A minor toe (usually the second) is flexed at the proximal interphalangeal joint and hyperextended at the distal inter-

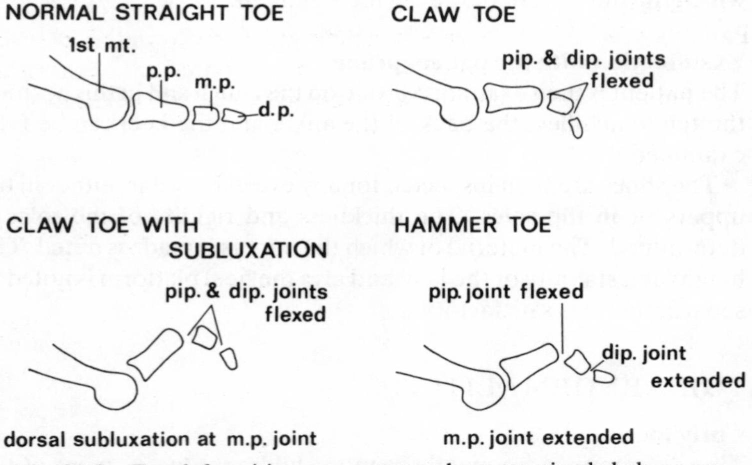

Fig. 21.8   Toe deformities: mt, metatarsal; pp, proximal phalanx; mp, middle phalanx; dp, distal phalanx; pip, proximal interphalangeal; dip, distal interphalangeal.

phalangeal joint. Patients complain of symptoms from shoe pressure over the proximal interphalangeal joint (Fig. 21.8d).

If the symptoms are significant, it is best to correct the deformity by arthrodesing the proximal interphalangeal joint.

Claw toes

Clawing of the minor toes occurs frequently in generalised diseases (Fig. 21.8b, c). It is seen in patients with rheumatoid arthritis and also seen in patients with neuromuscular diseases such as cerebral palsy or after strokes. The minor toes are flexed at the proximal and distal interphalangeal joints. The patients will complain of symptoms from shoe pressure. If the symptoms are significant, they can be corrected by operation. In a child, it is probably best to transfer the long flexor tendons into the extensor expansion. In an adolescent or mature patient, a more certain correction is obtained by arthrodesing both the distal and interphalangeal joints. In patients with rheumatoid arthritis, claw toes are usually associated with a subluxation or dislocation dorsally of the proximal phalanx at the metatarsophalangeal joint. In these patients, an excision arhroplasty excising both the metatarsal heads and the bases of the proximal phalanges (Fowler's operation) can give worthwhile relief.

Hallux valgus

Patients with this deformity have the great toe deviated laterally (Fig. 21.9). This deviation may be predisposed to by a varus alignment of the first metatarsal in relation to the rest of the foot. In

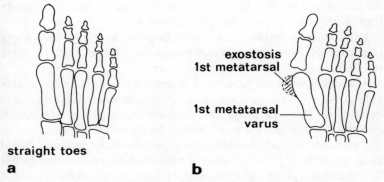

exostosis
1st metatarsal

1st metatarsal
varus

straight toes

a   **b**

Fig. 21.9 (a) Normal foot, (b) hallux valgus.

either case, the head of the first metatarsal becomes prominent on the medial side of the foot and subject to shoe pressure. As a result, an exostosis is formed with an overlying bursa. On occasions, this bursa becomes inflamed or even infected and is known as a bunion. Hallux valgus is a common deformity. It is also found in association with abnormalities of alignment of the metatarsal heads. In some cases, patients may have marked hallux valgus and complain of pain

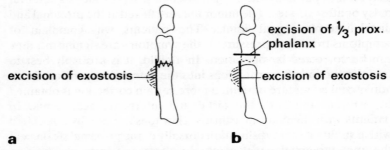

excision of exostosis

excision of ⅓ prox. phalanx

excision of exostosis

a   **b**

Fig. 21.10   (a) Arthrodesis of first metatarsophalangeal joint, (b) Keller's operation.

over the second or third metatarsal heads which are taking more weight than they should be. It is important to ascertain the site of the patient's pain so that appropriate treatment can be given.

Hallux valgus can be accentuated by tight fitting shoes, particularly in patients with metatarsus primus varus deformity. It is also seen in patients with rheumatoid arthritis of the foot. Gout frequently affects the first metatarsophalangeal joint and a gouty tophus may be similar to an infected bunion.

Patients with hallux valgus and bunions may be made more comfortable by wearing shoes adequate for the feet. In some patients, surgical shoes have to be made.

Various operations have been described for bunions and hallux valgus. A Keller's excision arthroplasty is one of the classical operations (Fig. 21.10b). The base of the proximal phalanx is excised to allow the toe to straighten by removing the insertion of the adductor hallucis tendon. The exostosis of the first metatarsal head is trimmed off. This leaves the patient with a mobile but rather flail and short, great toe. However, it is a very satisfactory operation in a great many patients. If there is an an excessive degree of varus of the first metatarsal, an osteotomy can be performed to correct this at the same time.

However, if a patient's main complaint is of pain under the second or third metatarsal, a Keller's operation may make this worse. A very adequate correction of the deformity can be obtained by arthrodesing the first metatarsophalangeal joint and removing the bunion (Fig. 21.10a). Care must be taken to set the great toe at the correct angle. The patient will have rigidity of this joint and will be unable to accommodate the foot to very high heels. However, they will have a strong pillar on the medial side of the foot, and this is the best operation for hallux valgus associated with metatarsalgia of any severity.

In adolescents and children, the hallux valgus is nearly always associated with a marked degree of metatarsus varus. This can be corrected by an osteotomy.

Hallux rigidus
Patients with this condition complain of a stiff and painful joint between the first metatarsal and the great toe. It is usually found in middle-aged people and radiographs show osteoarthritis of the metatarsophalangeal joint (Fig. 21.11). There may be an associated bunion. The symptoms can be relieved by wearing a shoe with a very firm sole or by fitting a metatarsal bar so that the strain is taken off the metatarsophalangeal joint. Sometimes the symptoms are so severe, the patient requires an operation. The operation of choice is to arthrodese the metatarsophalangeal joint and trim off any exostoses.

There is a condition known as juvenile hallux rigidus which is found in adolescent patients. These patients also complain of stiffness and pain of the metatarsophalangeal joint, and are found

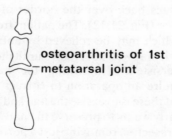

osteoarthritis of 1st
metatarsal joint

Fig. 21.11   Hallux rigidus.

to have marked limitation of dorsiflexion movement of the great toe at this joint.

Ingrowing great toe nail

This is a very common condition which causes quite distressing symptoms, particularly if the adjacent tissue becomes infected. The great toe nail tends to grow into the soft tissue at its margin. It may occur as a result of trauma or due to incorrect cutting of the nail.

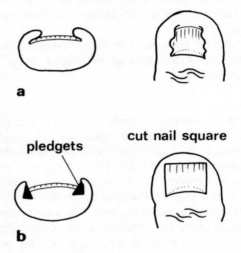

pledgets   **cut nail square**

Fig. 21.12   (a) Ingrowing toenail, (b) conservative treatment.

The patient should be advised to cut the nail straight across and also to roll the tissues back over the border of the nail using a pledget of silver paper (Fig. 21.12). The patient frequently presents with an infection which may be relieved by antibiotics and local measures. However it may well not resolve until the nail is avulsed.

Patients with persistently ingrowing toe nails, in spite of treatment, may require an operation to correct the abnormality. The most effective of these is to excise the nail and nail bed *in toto*. If the patient particularly wants to preserve the nail, then it is possible to perform a wedge resection removing just a portion of the nail and the base of the nail bed adjacent to it.

METATARSALGIA

Metatarsalgia is the term used for pain across the forefoot in the region of the metatarsal heads. It is a very frequent complaint and the causes (Fig. 21.13) include:

1. Malalignment of the metatarsal heads.
2. Rheumatoid arthritis (which may be early or late).
3. March fracture.
4. Freiberg's osteochondritis of a metatarsal head.
5. Morton's digital neuroma.
6. Lesions such as a ganglion or a lipoma.

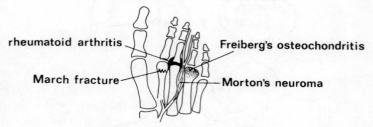

Fig. 21.13   Causes of metatarsalgia.

Malalignment of the metatarsal heads

This is probably the commonest cause of metatarsalgia (Fig. 21.14). The patient complains of pain across the metatarsal heads on weight bearing.

On examination, there are often callosities over the offending metatarsal heads and they can be seen and palpated to be more prominent than their neighbours. There may be associated abnormalities of the metatarsophalangeal joint such as dorsal subluxation of the proximal phalanx. There may be associated hallux valgus.

The patient's shoe should be inspected. The condition can be caused by crowding of the metatarsals in a shoe that is too tight across the forefoot. This crowding is frequently made worse when the patient has a high heel which tends to throw the majority of the weight onto the crowded metatarsal heads.

Acute symptoms can often be relieved by wearing comfortable shoes. Sometimes physiotherapy such as faradic foot baths gives very satisfactory relief. A metatarsal dome insole will relieve the

normal alignment of metatarsal heads all on the same horizontal plane

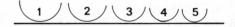

"dropping" of 2nd & 3rd metatarsal heads permitting unequal weight bearing

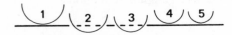

Fig. 21.14　Postural metatarsalgia.

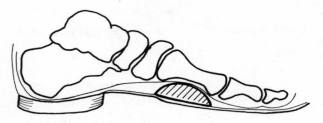

Fig. 21.15　Metatarsal dome insole.

weight over the metatarsal heads provided it is worn in a shoe with a low heel (Fig. 21.15). Very occasionally the symptoms are such that surgery is required and the 'dropped' metatarsals can be realigned by an osteotomy.

Rheumatoid arthritis

This may present with metatarsalgia. In these patients, the first joint affected is the metatarsophalangeal joint. There is a diffuse swelling in the region of the metatarsophalangeal joints of the foot and there will be tenderness around these joints. Other signs of rheumatoid arthritis may be noticed. At this stage, the X-ray is usually normal.

The treatment of these patients is that of the causative disease. The metatarsalgia may be relieved considerably by a dome insole.

Patients who have had rheumatoid arthritis for some time will develop deformities of the metatarsophalangeal joint. The minor toes become clawed and the proximal phalanx tends to sublux dorsally, on the metatarsal heads. These patients get intense pain from shoe pressure on walking.

On examination, the proximal phalanx can be felt to be subluxed or even dislocated and the metatarsal head is very prominent indeed on the sole of the foot. These patients can be relieved to some extent by specially made shoes which can accommodate the deformed toes. However an operation can be performed to relieve the condition which involves excising not only the metatarsal heads, but the proximal portion of the proximal phalanx leaving a false joint. In some patients with gross deformities and poor circulation in the foot, amputation of all the toes affords worthwhile relief of the symptoms.

March fracture

This occurs classically after a long walk on a hard road, by a person who is not used to such exercise. The next day, he develops intense pain in the region of the metatarsals. The original X-ray may be normal, and the lesion not diagnosed until a further X-ray is taken some weeks later, when a cloud of callus can be seen at the site of the stress fracture.

The condition is best treated by immobilisation in plaster, and the symptoms will rapidly resolve.

Freiberg's osteochondritis

This is an osteochondritis which occurs in the heads of the minor metatarsals. The patient complains of severe metatarsalgia. On examination, there is some irregularity and swelling of the metatarsal head affected. An X-ray will show the increased density and irregularity of the metatarsal head. These patients can be treated with a metatarsal dome insole. If the symptoms are acute, immobilisation in plaster may cause the symptoms to subside. If in spite of these measures the symptoms persist, it is reasonable to excise the metatarsal head by operation.

Morton's digital neuroma

The digital nerves bifurcate just proximal to the metatarsal heads and the transverse metatarsal ligament. At this bifurcation, a 'neuroma' can develop and cause intense metatarsalgia.

On examination, there is a discreetly tender area in the space between the metatarsal heads. In some cases, there may be associated hypo-aesthesia on the adjacent sides of the relevant toes.

This condition is best treated by excision of the neuroma when there will be dramatic relief of symptoms.

SYNOVITIS OF THE TIBIALIS POSTERIOR TENDON

Patients complain of pain at this site and there may be a sausage shaped swelling along the line of the tibialis posterior. There is pain on trying to perform inversion movements of the foot. The lesion may be seen in association with rheumatoid arthritis. It is best treated with rest, such as immobilisation in plaster. If there is a definite swelling with associated crepitus, it may be injected with local anaesthetic and steroids.

TENOSYNOVITIS OF THE PERONEAL TENDONS

Patients with this condition present in a similar fashion with pain over the outer side of the foot. There may be a sausage shaped swelling along the line of the peroneal tendons with crepitus on movement. The patient will complain of pain particularly on eversion.

This condition also can be treated with immobilisation in plaster. If there is a definite swelling, it can be injected with local anaesthetic and steroids.

DISLOCATION OF THE PERONEAL TENDONS

The tendons of peroneus longus and peroneus brevis pass into the foot behind the lateral malleolus and are held in place by a retinaculum.

For some reason, this may become damaged and the tendons can dislocate forward with an unpleasant painful clicking sensation.

Sometimes these symptoms are such that an operation is required. The retinaculum can be replaced by a fold of periosteum from the fibula.

RUPTURE OF THE TENDO ACHILLES

The tendo achilles becomes degenerate with age. A rupture is liable to occur through this degenerate portion. At operation, the tendon appears as a mass of degenerate fibrous tissue with clot or calcification interposed between the fibres. The patient complains of sudden pain in the back of the heel (as though being hit). It usually occurs whilst running or during sporting activity of some sort. On examination, the back of the lower leg is swollen. There may be a palpable gap in the tendo achilles. The 'squeeze test' may be positive. The patient lies prone with the foot just over the edge of the examination couch. Squeezing of the gastrocnemius-soleus complex in the normal leg will cause the foot to plantar flex. If the tendo achilles is ruptured, then there will be no such plantar flexion (Fig. 21.16).

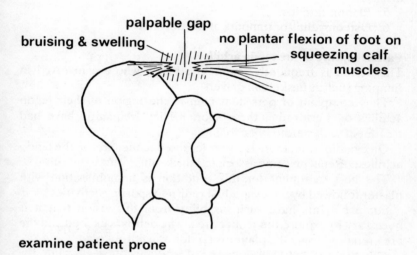

Fig. 21.16   Test for a ruptured tendo achilles.

The best results are obtained by performing an open operation. At operation, the clot and degenerative tissue is cleaned out and the ends of the tendon are approximated and sutured. The leg must be maintained in a below knee plaster with the foot plantar flexed for about seven or eight weeks after operation. It is possible to treat this lesion conservatively by immobilisation in a plaster with the foot plantar flexed for about eight weeks. In order to obtain good results by this method, it is necessary to immobilise the leg very soon after injury.

Patients frequently present late with this lesion. In such cases, the results of active treatment are not so satisfactory, and the residual disability may not be great.

PAINFUL HEEL LESIONS

Patients frequently complain of pain in the heel, particularly athletic patients. Some of the common causes are:
1. Partial rupture of tendo achilles.
2. Tendo achilles 'bursitis'.
3. Exostoses of the calcaneus.
4. Osteochondrosis of the epiphysis of the calcaneus (Sever's disease).
5. Plantar fasciitis.
6. Osteomyelitis or tumours of the calcaneus.

Partial rupture of the tendo achilles
This lesion is frequently found in athletes who are involved in jumping such as basketball players.

They complain of persistent pain in the region of their tendo achilles on performing these sports. They frequently have had treatment with steroid injections.

On examination, there is a very localised tender area in the tendo achilles, often with some associated thickening.

The best treatment for this condition is immobilisation with plaster followed by a very gradual return to sporting activities.

Some patients have such disability from this lesion that it is necessary to explore the tender area. The debris is excised and the area repaired using the plantaris tendon as a fibrous plait.

Tendo achilles 'bursitis'
There is no true tendon sheath around the tendo achilles, but there is an indefinite bursa. Athletic patients will quite frequently complain of pain in this area on running and jumping.

On examination, there is diffuse tenderness over the tendo achilles and, on occasions, some diffuse thickening. This condition is unsatisfactory to treat. Rest and immobilisation in plaster is followed by very gradual return to activities. In very resistant cases, the lesion can be explored and the thickened bursa removed.

Exostosis of the calcaneus
This may cause pain in the heel from shoe pressure. It is usually seen

in adolescents. They complain of a painful bony swelling at the posterolateral aspect of the calcaneus. On examination, there is a bony prominence at this site, and there may be some redness and swelling overlying it. The symptoms can be relieved by wearing soft shoes and in due course the symptoms will resolve. However, if the patient has persistent symptoms, the bony prominence can be excised.

Osteochondrosis of the epiphysis of the calcaneus (Sever's disease)
This condition occurs in athletic children such as young sprinters or jumpers. They complain of pain over the calcaneus at the insertion of the tendo achilles. On examination they are tender at this site. X-ray shows increased density and sometimes fragmentation of the epiphysis of the calcaneus.

This condition represents an osteochondrosis of the epiphysis of the calcaneus due to excessive traction of the tendo achilles.

The treatment is essentially conservative with rest and, if necessary, immobilisation in plaster.

(There is some doubt whether the above condition represents a specific disease process; however there is no doubt that patients frequently present with such signs and symptoms and that the condition will resolve with the treatment as outlined).

Plantar fasciitis
This condition occurs frequently in middle aged people who are overweight. They complain of pain under the heel at the site of the tubercle of the calcaneus to which the plantar fascia is attached.

On examination, there is tenderness in this region and X-ray may show a spur of the calcaneus. (This spur represents the result of the lesion rather than its cause.)

This lesion is best managed conservatively with advice as regards weight and wearing a pad in the shoe. If this fails, an injection of local anaesthetic and steroid is often effective. Occasionally the lesion is so resistant to treatment, an operation is carried out. This involves release not only of the insertion of the plantar fascia but also of the adjacent small muscles of the foot from the calcaneus.

A similar lesion is described in children and adolescents. In these patients, it is frequently associated with activity. They may also have a cavus foot. In these children, the best line of treatment is rest from activities and immobilising the foot in plaster.

Very occasionally they require an operation and a similar procedure to that in adults is performed.

LESIONS OF THE ANKLE JOINT

Osteoarthritis of the ankle joint

This condition usually occurs after injuries such as fractures or severe ligament injuries. It is also seen following infectious arthritis or rheumatoid arthritis.

The ankle joint is a weight bearing joint. Patients with osteoarthritis of the ankle joint often have such severe symptoms that operative treatment is required. They complain of persistent pain or swelling around the ankle with diminution in the range of movements. These symptoms are worse on weight bearing.

On examination, there is tenderness around the ankle joint line. There may be associated swelling in this region. The range of movements is markedly reduced. X-ray will show narrowing of the joint space and sclerosis of the underlying bone. If the original lesion was a fracture or ligament injury, incongruity of the ankle joint may be seen.

Conservative treatment involves the use of physiotherapy and anti-inflammatory drugs. If the symptoms are more severe, a weight relieving caliper may be necessary

Operation is commonly required for osteoarthritis of the ankle. The operation usually performed is an arthrodesis. The ankle joint is fused in about ten degrees of equinus in relation to the leg. If there is good function of the subtalar joint, a very reasonable result is obtained (Fig. 21.17). Recently an ankle prosthesis has been developed and some good results are obtained from this (particularly in patients with rheumatoid arthritis).

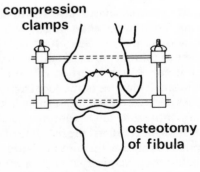

compression clamps

osteotomy of fibula

Fig. 21.17 Ankle arthrodesis.

Footballer's ankle

Footballers frequently complain of pain over the anterior aspect of the ankle. There may be tenderness at this site, limitation of plantar flexion movement and associated swelling.

X-ray shows some irregularity over the superior aspect of the neck of the talus. The best treatment is rest with restriction of activities. This is followed by graduated exercise and eventually return to playing football.

In some cases, the symptoms are so persistent, that an operation is required to excise the bony masses of the neck of the talus.

Chronic instability of the lateral ligament

The commonest injury about the ankle is the inversion sprain. In this lesion, the fibres of the anterolateral ligament of the ankle are disrupted. These usually heal with rest.

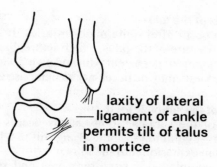

laxity of lateral ligament of ankle permits tilt of talus in mortice

Fig. 21.18   Lateral ligament instability.

The lateral ligament itself consists of three portions, the posterior talo-fibular portion, the portion between the fibula and the tubercle of the calcaneus, and the anterior portion of the ligament. If these are disrupted and not allowed to heal, some laxity of the lateral ligament results.

These patients complain of persistent giving way of the ankle particularly on playing sport. On examination, there is tenderness over the outer side of the ankle. There is increased mobility of the foot and ankle on forced inversion (Fig. 21.18).

It is best to treat a severe sprain of the ankle with a below knee plaster for three or four weeks. If this is performed as a routine on all those patients who cannot bear weight after such an injury, a great number of these injuries to the lateral ligament will heal spontaneously with little residual disability.

Patients with persistent symptoms can be managed conservatively. This involves special exercises; an outside float to the heel can be tried. Some patients have such severe symptoms that a caliper such as a polypropylene splint or an iron with an outside T strap can be used. Active patients however often require operative treatment. The diagnosis should be confirmed by performing a stress X-ray under general anaesthetic. The lateral ligament is stressed on the affected side and also on the normal foot. AP X-rays are taken of both feet in the fully inverted position. When chronic laxity of the lateral ligament is present, the talus will tilt markedly on inversion.

At operation, the peroneus bevis tendon is used, and is threaded along the line of the lateral ligament and also between the talus and the lateral malleolus.

Osteochondritis of the talus
This lesion can occur after quite minor injuries. It is probably an osteochondral fracture of the talus. The fracture does not heal and the patient complains of persistent pain and giving way of the ankle. Special oblique views may be necessary to demonstrate the lesion.

Osteoarthritis of the subtalar joint
Osteoarthritis of the subtalar joint usually occurs as a result of trauma. The most common lesion causing this is a fracture of the calcaneus with an extension into the joint.

The patient complains of persistent pain and stiffness in the months after fracture. Instead of the symptoms resolving, they become more severe and more persistent as osteoarthritis develops.

These patients can be managed conservatively by a polypropylene splint to control inversion and eversion movements of the subtalar joint. If this fails, then an operation can be performed to arthrodese the subtalar joint.

In patients who have fractures of the calcaneus, the joint between the calcaneus and the cuboid is often damaged as well as that between the talus and the calcaneus. It is probably best to perform a triple arthrodesis for these patients (Fig. 21.19).

Rheumatoid arthritis of the subtalar joint
Rheumatoid arthritis often affects the subtalar joint. Patients complain of swelling in the region of the sinus tarsi which can be palpated just anterior to the lateral malleolus. There is pain on

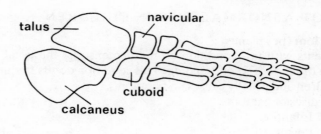

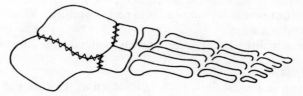

Fig. 21.19   Triple arthrodesis of foot.

stressing the subtalar joint and this pain occurs particularly on walking on rough ground.

Treatment is similar to that of osteoarthritis. Operation when required can usually be confined to the subtalar joint. A graft can be used with a very worthwhile relief of symptoms.

Arthritis of the midtarsal joint

Arthritis of the midtarsal joint occurs particularly in patients with foot deformities. Patients with flat foot may have deformity for a great many years without symptoms and then eventually develop pain from arthritis in middle life. X-rays will show degenerative changes in the joints affected. These patients can be managed conservatively with a firm valgus insole. This will support the longitudinal arch. Acute symptoms can be relieved by physiotherapy and anti-inflammatory drugs.

Osteochondrosis of the navicular (Kohler's disease)

This condition occurs in young children who present with limp and pain in the foot. X-ray shows sclerosis and fragmentation of the navicular. These patients can be treated with a plaster cast which will resolve the symptoms rapidly. The navicular usually heals and returns to normal in due course.

FOOT ABNORMALITIES IN CHILDREN

Flat foot (pes planus)

Patients with this condition do not demonstrate the usual medial arch of the foot when standing. This condition occurs frequently in children and usually causes no symptoms.

Causes of flat foot:
1. Infantile.
2. Postural.
3. Tight tendo achilles (as in cerebral palsy).
4. Neuromuscular imbalance (as in poliomyelitis).
5. Tarsal coalition.
6. Abnormalities of the forefoot such as metatarsus adductus.

Infantile flat foot

This is seen in practically all young children as they start to walk. There is a considerable amount of fibro fatty tissue which obliterates the arch. In due course, the foot will develop normally with no treatmnt.

Postural flat foot

This is seen in older children with persistent flat foot associated with a valgus heel.

The longitudinal arch is to some extent dependent on the position of the subtalar joint and the reciprocal motion of the metatarsals. Inversion movement of the subtalar joint combined with flexion movement of the first metatarsal will cause the arch to be raised in the weight bearing foot. Eversion movement at the subtalar joint combined with a reciprocal extension movement of the first metatarsal will cause the arch to flatten in the weight bearing foot.

The subtalar joint acts as an oblique hinge and during weight bearing, movements of the subtalar joint are coupled to rotary movements which occur in the lower limb. External rotation movements of the lower limb will be accompanied by inversion of the subtalar joint (which will raise the arch of the foot). Internal rotation movements of the lower limb will be coupled with eversion movement of the subtalar joint (which will lower the arch of the foot) (Fig. 21.20 and 21.21).

In young children, the extensors and external rotators of the hip tend to lag behind in function during development, so that the lower limb tends to 'slump' into internal rotation with a reciprocal eversion of the subtalar joint and lowering of the arch of the foot.

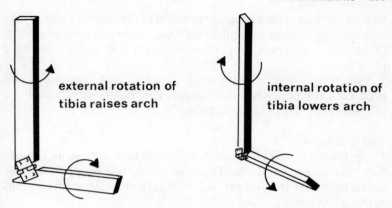

external rotation of tibia raises arch

internal rotation of tibia lowers arch

Fig. 21.20 Subtalar joint as an oblique hinge.

As part of normal development, this slump will in due course be alleviated. However in certain children, in particular those with neuromuscular defects, it tends to persist. If flat foot persists, the foot is liable to become rigid in the flat foot position. It can no longer be corrected. Fortunately, people with such flat foot usually remain symptom-free. The majority of young children with postural flat foot will return to normal in due course. It is reasonable to fit them with an inside wedge on the heel of their shoe extending onto the sole. This will protect the shoe against excessive wear.

However, in an older child, if the lesion is persistent it can be corrected by using a plastic heel cup with an extension on the inner

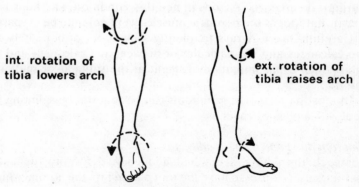

int. rotation of tibia lowers arch

ext. rotation of tibia raises arch

Fig. 21.21 Arch and rotation of leg.

side of the foot. This is used as an insert in the ordinary shoe. Very occasionally, in the older child (aged eight to twelve), an osteotomy of the calcaneus may be performed to push it into the inverted position.

Sometimes, particularly with patients with neuromuscular problems, it is necessary to arthrodese the subtalar joint wedging it into inversion with a block of bone.

Tendo achilles

Patients who have tight tendo achilles will tend to have an equinus foot. In order to get the heel into the weight bearing position, they find it necessary to evert the foot fully at the subtalar joint and thus causing a flattening of the arch.

All children with flat foot should be checked for a tight tendo achilles. If it is tight, it can be stretched by a physiotherapist, or if this fails, a simple operation can be performed to lengthen the tendon and permit correction of the deformity.

Neuromuscular flat foot

This occurs in conditions causing neuromuscular imbalance such as poliomyelitis, meningomyelocele and cerebral palsy. It is theoretically possible to correct this by doing tendon transfers, but in practice, it is usually found necessary to perform an arthrodesis of the subtalar joint wedging it into inversion. This of course can only be performed satisfactorily on the older child.

Flat foot due to tarsal coalition

These patients tend to present with flat foot which becomes painful during adolescence. At one time, this condition was known as spastic flat foot as the peroneal muscles were noted to be in spasm.

Carefully taken X-rays frequently show a bar of bone between the calcaneus and the navicular or between the calcaneus and the talus. Such a bar impairs movement at the subtalar or midtarsal joints.

In most patients, the symptoms can be relieved by splinting the heel with a plastic heel cup.

Flat foot due to metatarsus adductus

Some children have a residual adduction deformity of all the metatarsals. In order to have the foot placed into the normal weight bearing position, it is necessary for the metatarsals to twist outwards and this will cause a secondary eversion movement at the subtalar joint. The arch will thus be lowered, and secondary flat foot results.

Intoe gait
Young children frequently walk with an intoe gait. The causes are:
1. Postural abnormalities.
2. Metatarsus adductus.
3. Tibial torsion.
4. Femoral neck anteversion.
5. Neuromuscular disorders.

Postural abnormalities
Young children frequently start to walk with an intoe gait. These children also tend to have flat feet with everted heels. In due course, this will correct itself without treatment.

If the shoes are worn down excessively on the inner side, then it is reasonable to wedge the heel and extend it onto the sole to improve the shoe wear.

Metatarsus adductus (adducted forefoot)
These children have a forefoot which is adducted on the hind foot, so that it appears banana shaped. The hind foot is usually normal and the heel appears straight (Fig. 21.22).

This condition improves with simple treatment. Continuous pressure on the adducted forefoot can be applied by putting the shoes on the opposite feet. If this fails, plasters can be applied, and if they are put on under anaesthetic, it is possible to manipulate the foot gently at the same time. If the lesion persists after the age of six or seven, it is possible to do an osteotomy of the bases of the metatarsal bones to correct the deformity.

Quite often, children who have been treated for club foot have a residual adduction of the metatarsals. These children frequently have an inversion abnormality of the heel as well.

Tibial torsion
The ankle joint is normally aligned so that it deviates laterally at ten degrees to the long axis of the tibia. In these children, the foot is either pointing straight forward, or twisted inwards on the tibia. It is sometimes seen with a bow leg deformity.

This condition also will resolve itself spontaneously. If it is marked, then a splint may be used to correct it. A useful splint is the

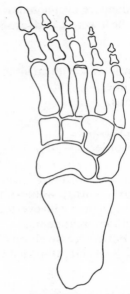

Fig. 21.22   Metatarsus adductus.

Dennis Browne splint to use at night. The feet are applied to the plate in external rotation. Very rarely the deformity is such that it requires an osteotomy to correct it.

Femoral neck anteversion (see Fig. 19.14, p. 191)
This condition occurs quite frequently in children. The femoral neck tends to point forwards instead of in the normal coronal plane. As a result, the children tend to internally rotate the lower limb in order to accommodate the head of the femur more efficiently in the acetabulum.

On examination, the children will intoe. The patellae will tend to point inwards. When the children sit, they tend to sit with their hips in internal rotation, and their legs on either side of the buttocks (the so-called television position). On examination of the hip joint, it will be found that there is an increased range of internal rotation and a decreased range of external rotation movement.

Fortunately, this condition tends to resolve itself spontaneously. If the shoe is worn excessively on the inner side, it is reasonable to use a small inside raise on the heel extending onto the sole. In severe cases, it is sometimes worthwhile using a heel cup to hold the heel in inversion and thus externally rotate the lower limb. Very rarely, children with a severe deformity require an osteotomy to correct it.

Femoral neck anteversion may be associated with congenital dislocation of the hip as a secondary abnormality. Children presenting with an intoe gait should have an X-ray of the hips to exclude this.

Neuromuscular causes of the intoe gait

Neuromuscular lesions can produce an imbalance about the hip, particularly in patients with cerebral palsy or with meningo-myelocele. This imbalance can produce an intoe gait. Treatment of intoe gait in these patients involves correction of the neuromuscular imbalance.

TALIPES EQUINOVARUS (club foot)

Children with this condition are born with the foot twisted inwards (Fig. 21.23). The heel is tight and inverted and the forefoot adducted. This position is produced by a severe equinus contracture, in addition there is severe varus contracture at the subtalar joint, and marked adduction deformity of the forefoot on the hind foot.

The condition occurs in about one per thousand births. It is frequently associated with other abnormalities such as cleft palate and congenital dislocation of the hip and is seen as part of the complex of arthrogryphosis. There is an increased family incidence.

In order to obtain adequate correction, it demands treatment as soon as possible after birth. The position is held by contracted fibrous tissue on the inner side and the back of the foot. If the child is permitted to develop with this deformity uncorrected, in due course the bones of the foot will develop an abnormal shape and perpetuate the deformity. Initial treatment involves persistent gentle manipulation followed by splintage by strapping, plaster or a Dennis Browne splint.

A Dennis Browne splint consists of a foot plate; bolted to this are two vertical projections. The feet are strapped to the vertical projections so that the soles are as flat as possible on the foot plate. As the child kicks, it will tend to spontaneously correct the feet with a series of self-induced manipulations.

A certain percentage of childen with club feet can be reduced and

FRONT
feet inverted

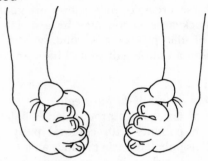

BACK

thin calves

tight inverted heels

adducted forefeet

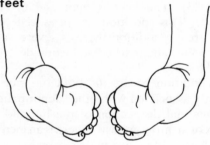

Fig. 21.23   Club foot.

held corrected by such conservative measures. After treatment with manipulation and splintage, night splints should be worn for at least one year. When the child starts to walk, his shoe should have an outside raise and he should be kept under observation for several years as the condition has a tendency to relapse.

However, the greater proportion of children with club feet do not obtain an adequate correction with such conservative measures. Early operation is required. At operation, all the tight tissues on the inner side and the posterior aspect of the foot are divided. This includes the tendons of the tibialis posterior and flexor digitorum longus and the tendo achilles is lengthened. All the ligaments on the posterior and medial aspect of the foot are divided so that the talus is practically freed from the rest of the foot.

Having done this, it is possible to place the foot on the talus in the desired position. Position is held for some months, and splints are worn for some months afterwards.

In spite of this, patients present in later life with persistent deformities from club foot. These include an equinus deformity, or a varus of the heel, or an adduction of the forefoot.

In later life, patients require bony operations to correct these deformities. The most effective of these is the triple arthrodesis. This involves taking a wedge of bone from the joint between the calcaneus and the cuboid and the joint between the navicular and the talus. By doing this, practically any deformity of the foot may be corrected, but the foot is left rigid and rather small. This operation cannot be effectively performed before the age of twelve or thirteen (see Fig. 21.19).

Further Reading

AEGERTER E. & KIRKPATRICK J. (1975) *Orthopedic Diseases: Physiology, Pathology and Radiology*, 4th ed. Philadelphia: W. B. Saunders.

Aids to the Examination of the Peripheral Nervous System (1976) Medical Research Council Memorandum No. 45. London: HMSO.

AMERICAN ACADEMY OF ORTHOPEDIC SURGEONS (1966) *Joint Motion, Method of Measuring and Recording*. Edinburgh: Churchill Livingstone.

AMERICAN ACADEMY OF ORTHOPEDIC SURGEONS (1975) *Atlas of Orthotics: Biomechanical Principles and Applications*. St Louis: C. V. Mosby.

CRAWFORD ADAMS J. (1976) *Outline of Orthopaedics*, 8th ed. Edinburgh: Churchill Livingstone.

EDMONSON A. S. & CRENSHAW M. D. (1980) *Campbell's Operative Orthopaedics*, 6th ed. St Louis: C. V. Mosby.

FROST H. M. (1973) *Orthopaedic Biomechanics*. Orthopaedic Lectures Vol. 5. Springfield, Illinois: Charles C. Thomas.

HOPENFELDT S. (1977) *Orthopaedic Neurology, A Diagnostic Guide to Neurological Levels*. Philadelphia: J. B. Lippencott.

MCNAB I. (1977) *Backache*. Baltimore: Williams & Wilkins.

MOSELEY H. F. (1969) *Shoulder Lesions*, 3rd ed. Edinburgh: Churchill Livingstone.

RANG M. (1967) *The Growth Plate and its Disorders*. Edinburgh: Churchill Livingstone.

SMILLIE I. S. (1978) *Injuries of the Knee Joint*, 5th ed. Edinburgh: Churchill Livingstone.

WYNNE-DAVIES R. & FAIRBANK T. J. (1976) *Fairbank's Atlas of General Affections of the Skeleton*, 2nd ed. Edinburgh: Churchill Livingstone.

Index

267